Praise for *BARREN – The Inside World of Infertility*

"*Barren - The Inside World of Infertility* is a riveting look at the struggles couples face when they decide to pursue fertility treatment. The book is very beautifully written and organized. It helps the readers understand the various types of treatment couples or individuals must undertake when they decide to see a fertility specialist.

The individual memoirs in Part Two truly bring home the emotional roller coasters both men and women endure when faced with the challenges of becoming parents through fertility treatment and help the readers to not only understand the diagnoses and treatment options, but the hidden costs that the individuals experience when going through fertility treatment.

Infertility is a taboo, and most couples do not share the struggles they faced trying to conceive or needing to consider fertility treatment. This makes their journey very lonely and the feeling of hopelessness and despair inevitable.

Barren is the first book everyone having difficulty conceiving or is considering fertility treatment should read. The book breaks down all the types of treatment options that are available from least aggressive to the most aggressive treatment including IVF and third-party reproduction with donor eggs, donor sperm, donor embryos, and surrogacy.

Pamela Rasheed has truly pulled the curtain back on the inside world of infertility for all to see and understand. As a fertility doctor, *Barren - The Inside World of Infertility* is a book that I will recommend to all my patients. This is a must read for anyone having difficulty conceiving as well as for their family members, friends, and clinicians."

– *Dr. Melvin Thornton* – Reproductive Endocrinologist. New York and Connecticut

"*Barren* is a wonderfully written, comprehensive and insightful book about the oftentimes difficult subject of infertility. Not only does the author take you inside the diagnoses, medicine, and cutting-edge technology and interventions to overcome infertility, but exposes the raw emotions and personal struggles women and their partners face on this difficult path. This book is an absolute read for anyone considering the long and daunting journey of in-vitro fertilization. I especially appreciate the personal experiences of the numerous couples who are profiled in this publication. Pamela deserves much praise for her extensive knowledge and understanding of infertility and how she explains the process in significant detail."

– *Dr. Jay Matut*, OB-GYN, New York

"Beautifully written, Pamela Rasheed's book bridges the gaps between medicine, personal experiences, and practical knowledge. The subject of infertility is complicated and often very painful on a personal level. Ms. Rasheed does an excellent job exploring the many aspects of infertility with compassion and clarity. As an OB-GYN practicing medicine for over 30 years, and also as someone who worked with Ms. Rasheed, and I can vouch not only for her thorough understanding of fertility issues, but also her sincere empathy with patients. This is a well-researched book filled with useful information that should be considered essential reading for anyone struggling with infertility."

– *Dr. Kay. D. Anderson* – OB-GYN, New York and Florida

"Insightful, emotional, and eye opening: In this collection of memoirs, Pamela Rasheed gives readers an inside look into the complex and emotional world of infertility. *Barren* captures the raw, real-life experiences of women and couples navigating infertility and sheds light on important women's health issues and the hidden costs of infertility that are not nearly talked about enough. Drawing from her own experience as a fertility nurse, Pamela Rasheed breaks down the complexities of infertility treatments and medicine, and what I found to be particularly interesting is the component of preimplantation genetic testing technology. If you are battling infertility yourself or know someone who is, you will almost certainly learn something new from this book and will leave with a newfound empathy for all those struggling."

–Steve Chapman, CEO, Natera, Inc.

"The readers of this book are truly fortunate to have Pamela Rasheed, RN, share her knowledge of the IVF process. She has demystified the complexity of this innovative medical wonder. Her book gives readers all sides of the IVF experience that they will encounter: the medical, financial, and emotional challenges, the successes, and failures. Essentially, she is the coach, and this book is the manual for the IVF marathon.

My husband and I navigated these challenges on our own through the knowledge and wisdom our life experiences have taught us. We made mistakes and choices that were not perfect. An instructional book like this would have been beneficial to prevent and overcome our mistakes, insecurities, and fears along the way. Blessed with two miracle babies, I genuinely do not know if our IVF journey could have gone very wrong due to our lack of knowledge like most stories that I have heard. We were fortunate that we had Pamela on our team, who helped us prevent and fix some of our mistakes but finding our way to helpful hands was a lonely road."

— Jill Hudson, New York

"*Barren: The Inside World of Infertility* is an inside view from a brilliant nurse who has spent the most part of her career integrally involved in treating patients in one of the best fertility clinics in the world – Columbia University Fertility Center. This book is written in simple language catering for all cross-sections of readers. It offers detailed descriptions of diagnoses, treatments, and examines the mental preparation process for treatment through the experiences of several real-life stories of couples with infertility problems and issues.

Infertility is taboo and patients are left alone to figure out complex issues mostly understood by trained medical professionals. The biological complexities from the perspective of the lay person are often not simple but this author uses simple language to highlight the important factors from diagnoses to a successful treatment outcome. Nurse Pamela masterfully offers tips to navigating the complex layers of infertility including the pandemic and gives an all-round picture of what is most needed to be understood before starting a fertility treatment program.

And what is most downplayed in almost all treatment regimens by even the best hospitals and clinics is the hidden cost of infertility which is expertly introduced through the experiences of real patients. The stigma, grief, shame, fear and uncertainty, financial implications, spiritual, psychological, moral, and ethical impacts are brought to the forefront for mentally preparing couples who will be undertaking the journey of fertility treatment.

This book is most helpful to everyone having difficulties conceiving, and fertility facilities that often leave out of their care plans the mental and psychological effects their patients endured. This book is also a smart tool for undergrads, gynecologists, policy makers, and constitutional bodies who are preparing to draft legislation on fertility treatment, and anyone seeking information about infertility, treatment, and its hidden costs."

– *Valmiki Bankay* – Economist, Guyana, South America

"This book is an incredible account of all the challenges that impact couples with infertility issues. The stories are captivating with so many details of how infertility and pregnancy failure affected their lives. Pamela is amazing in pointing out the small unknown issues that arise when considering options to infertility. *Barren – The Inside World of Infertility* is a must read for not only couples with infertility issues but also for their loved ones, their support systems, and healthcare providers to better understand the emotional impact of infertility."

– *Laura A. Conklin*, MSN, MSA, RN, LNCC, CNE - Conklin and Associates, LLC

"It is important for patients to be forthcoming in their endeavors to fruitful parenthood and in this current day, there are so much information to serve as a guide for anyone who is willing to listen. Keep in mind that every "BODY" is different, and what might or might not have worked for one person will not be the same for everyone else. Having all that modern AND traditional medicinal technology can offer in one place certainly can make the journey much easier.

This book is like the Google Maps from "current location" to "destination"! The entire map is displayed for you, as well as route options. It is ultimately your choice which way to go, but regardless of the way, you can use it to "center" yourself to your surroundings to never lose sight of where you are on your path.

As a licensed practitioner of Acupuncture and TCM, the most helpful portion of this book, and any other book, is the Table of Contents: it is THE place to go to, regardless of whether you have read the entire book. It allows you the freedom to be in control of what information you feel ready to receive, vs. being locked in on a path that might not be the right one for me.

I would recommend this book to ANYONE, who is ready, and willing to learn what is out there that could be helpful. Just like my business: I run my practice with available office hours to try and help those who WANT my help. I cannot force anyone to come see me, nor would that be the right attitude to having when raising kids! The entire universe is like a mirror - the energy you put out will eventually be reflected to you."

– *Dr. Heebae Kong, L.Ac.*, Holistic Medicine – New York

"Infertility is an all-encompassing issue that affects women and couples physically, emotionally, and financially, and is an incredibly difficult world to navigate. With many years of experience as a nurse in the field of infertility, Pamela guides you through this challenging time. Her book goes through the basics, including diagnosing fertility issues and the common steps taken throughout the treatment process. She shares encouraging stories from those who have endured the highs and lows of this roller coaster ride. Pamela stresses the need for what might possibly be the single most important aspect for navigating this time — emotional support — and gives suggestions on how to obtain this from various sources. She talks about the benefits of incorporating alternative treatments, such as acupuncture, herbs, and massage therapy in addition to traditional Assisted Reproductive Technologies, and how they can ease stress and greatly improve outcomes.

I highly recommend this book for anyone brand new to the world of infertility, as well as for anyone who has been on their infertility journey for a long time. All those struggling with infertility deserve access to the knowledge and wisdom that this book imparts."

– *Roberta Klein-Siegelson* MS, L. Ac., South Shore Acupuncture and Fertility Wellness

"'Barren' — What does that word really mean? A question asked early in the book. It is a word that stirs up intense pain and confusion for many people. Several patients shared their journey and pointed out the support of a caring fertility team, which is imperative to successfully navigate the options to resolve being childless.

The end goal was self-healing from being barren with the potential hope of family building.

The author of this book turns the pain into hope and has tackled the subject in a constructive manner. This book is truly a road map to better understand infertility: the emotional, financial, spiritual costs, and the available treatment options.

This book is written for both the interfertile population and the professionals who desire to work in this field of infertility. It navigates us through early diagnosis, treatments options, and all the emotions that some must endure to building a family.

The more compassionate caring professionals who speak up and speak out to explain the stigma and taboo of being barren, the better chance to de-stigmatize this diagnosis.

By eradicating the stigma of infertility treatment through pure understanding, the better chance there is of making what is unbearable, possible! Pick up your copy today and become more hopeful."

— *Sylvia T. Parrett*, RN, MSW.

"Pamela Rasheed provides exactly the information and empathy infertile couples crave. The practical material outlines the options and procedures clearly. The real–life patients' stories highlight the persistence and emotional and psychological stamina needed for this roller coaster ride. I was in their shoes thirty-five years and two wonderful adult children ago, before a book like this existed. I highly recommend it for those seeking useful advice and compassion for those on the journey of infertility to parenthood."

— *Susan V. Haibeck* RN MS CLNC. President - Haibeck and Associates Legal Nurse Consulting

"This book offers an in-depth knowledge about diagnoses, available treatment options, and the downplayed hidden emotional, psychological, and financial costs involved in the infertility world. Also, the author's personal experience as a specialized registered nurse in this field touches your soul, offering hope to couples who are desperate and have almost given up. In addition to her step-by-step instructions, guidance, and support, couples can embrace a holistic approach to this type of treatment and the various avenues of assistance less considered previously.

This book proves that miracles can still happen, and I highly recommend it to those on this journey to parenthood (despite the difficulties), the clinicians who treat them, and their support teams."

— *Sharon Hans*

"*Barren – The Inside World of Infertility* gives the lay person and the professional healthcare provider a true inside look into the heart-felt problems that can arise from infertility in women and men.

Pamela Rasheed, RN, explains the medical aspects of all the different infertility treatments as well as the costs and insurance coverage in a manner that everyone can understand. The feelings of guilt and lack of understanding that women and men go through when they learn that they have difficulty conceiving are explained in this book.

Demonstrations of these feeling are presented through true stories of patients who have undergone infertility problems. Some of these patients finally conceived through various treatment options including donated gametes while others utilized the surrogacy and adoption pathways.

These stories place the reader in the shoes of the couples who have suffered disappointment, stigma, grief, shame, and uncertainty. The stress caused by financial costs without insurance can cause destruction of a family, especially when multiple treatments are done without success.

Barren is a must read for anyone who is having difficulty getting pregnant and those who are in their path to offer support. This book gives hope and understanding to those still trying to conceive. It is also a must read for healthcare providers who treat women and/or men with trouble starting a family. As a healthcare provider, myself, I think that we can become too complacent and less understanding when our patients become frustrated and depressed. This book emphasizes the need for healthcare providers to be understanding and even offer support groups so that our patients do not feel alone and misunderstood."

– *Melanie L. Balestra*, NP, ESQ

BARREN

―The Inside World of Infertility―

Pamela G. Rasheed,
MSN, RN

BARREN – The Inside World of Infertility

Copyright 2021 by Pamela G. Rasheed

Layout by Douglas Williams

Editorial support by Pat Iyer

Except as printed under the United States Copyright Act of 1976, no parts of this book may be reproduced or distributed in any form or by any means or stored in a database or retrieval system, without the prior written permission of the author. If you would like to quote from or otherwise use materials from this book, please contact the author at prasheed1@icloud.com

ISBN: 9798589400526

DEDICATION

This book is dedicated to the men and women who shared their stories in this book and to those who are still on this path.

You are brave, courageous, and strong despite the difficult and often lonely terrain of your specific fertility journey. Many of you have come to know the purest joy of parenthood and are bold enough to share your struggles and how you've overcome so that the others can be encouraged and know that miracles still happen.

Courage does not always roar.
Sometimes courage is the quiet voice at the end of the day saying,
"I will try again tomorrow"

–MARY ANNE RADMACHER

ACKNOWLEDGMENTS

This book would not be possible without the contribution of some of my patients' true stories, and I want to thank each of you. I want to also thank Dustin Moore and his wife Caren for sharing their beautiful adoption story. They shaped the depth of their experiences in the pages of this book.

I want to thank Dr. Melvin Thornton, Reproductive Endocrinologist, who served as the Medical Director of the Third-party Program at Columbia University - Center for Women's Reproductive Care (CWRC) during part of my tenure. He was responsible for my assignment as the head nurse in this division and was one of my mentors.

I want to thank my long-time friend, Valmiki Bankay, for his encouragement to write this book first. Valmiki is a graduate of the University of Guyana, an Economist, Agriculturist, Businessman, and a voice of reason when I pondered which book to write first.

A big thank you to the President of the National Nurses Business Association (NNBA), Michelle Podlesni, RN, speaker, and author of *Conventional Nurse*, who, at our very first meeting in 2017, stated, "I see a book in you." Words are powerful!

Thank you to my friends, Sophie Messan, a social worker who labored with me in the third-party program at Columbia University CWRC, Sylvia Parrett, RN, Jill Geldbach, and Sharon Hans, for their honest and consistent encouragement throughout this project.

Thanks to Cystic Fibrosis of New Zealand (CFNZ) for granting permission to use an image on their site related to autosomal recessive gene mutations.

My deepest gratitude to my two kids, Sarah Z. Rasheed, and Amir D. Rasheed, for being excellent in every way and for just being there during the hectic years of my studies and career development. They are my constant reminder of the joy and fulfillment of motherhood.

A thank you to my mother, Drupatie Baichanpersaud, for her silent approval in every chapter of my professional and personal journey.

Finally, to my editor and writing coach, Pat Iyer, RN, MSN, LNCC, author, editor, public speaker, and the best in the field of book mastery who provided the dedicated guidance necessary to bring this book to fruition. Thank you for turning the raw transcript into an amazing and inspirational book!

ABOUT THE AUTHOR

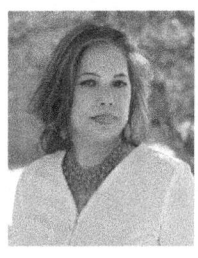
Pamela G. Rasheed is a registered nurse with a Master's degrees in the Science of Nursing and a pre-requisite Bachelor's degree in the Science of Nursing. She is a graduate of the City University of New York (CUNY) and Western Governors University in Utah. Pamela has an extensive background in women's health with more than a decade in the field of Reproductive Endocrinology (Infertility).

Pamela is presently employed as a Nurse Care Manager at The Women's Integrated Network (WIN), a national leader in Infertility Management Programs. In this role, she authorizes treatment plans and medications for various assisted reproductive technology (ART) protocols and provides extensive patient education and nursing support to the population with infertility.

As the founder and CEO of Gentle-Nurse Infusion, Pamela directs this private organization to provide services related to self-injections and intravenous (IV) infusion procedures, coaching, and nursing support specific to infertility treatments and procedures.

Before her current position, Pamela spent ten years at the prestigious Columbia University's Center of Women's Reproductive Care in New York City. As the medical assistant's department manager, she hired, trained, and evaluated medical assistants to provide the highest standard of reproductive patient care, including phlebotomy and other infertility related procedures, while emphasizing the importance of meeting the patients' needs and expectations.

As part of her tenure at Columbia University Medical Center, Pamela provided services in the position as RN-Officer of Administration, where she worked closely with the country's top reproductive endocrinologists managing infertility treatment protocols. Pamela managed patients' treatment protocols using autologous oocytes (patients' own eggs), donor eggs, and donor embryos for CWRC's clients in the USA and overseas.

Prior to entering the field of reproductive endocrinology in 2008, Pamela spent nine years in the field of Obstetrics and Gynecology (OB-GYN) as the clinical supervisor for medical assistants at the West-Care OB-GYN in NYC and Women's HealthCare OB-GYN in Westchester County.

Before migrating to the USA, Pamela spent two years as an elementary school teacher and subsequently as medical laboratory technician and medical assistant for four additional years at a notable private medical practice in Guyana.

Pamela is a member of the American Nurses Association (ANA), NY State Nurses Association (NYSNA), and the National Nurses in Business Association (NNBA). She is a graduate of The Assembly of God Bible College in Guyana and currently serves as a teacher in the Bible Institute of the Highland Church in Queens, New York. Pamela is a mother of two college-age children and lives on Long Island, New York.

Preface

I decided to write this book to bring to center stage the private non-medical struggles of the infertile population. Stigma, shame, blame, grief, secrecy, and other undiagnosed elements are ignored or shifted behind curtains because they are too private to expose.

My infertility nurse's book provides enlightenment about the challenges many patients face in infertility and how they navigate this hidden emotional and psychological pain in the medical diagnosis and treatment of infertility.

The infertile woman often turns to no one else but to the woman in the mirror and her nurse – if he or she is compassionate – to share disappointment and grief. As a result of the support I offered to infertile couples, we created a beautiful nurse-patient relationship and bonded throughout their journey and beyond with photographic updates of their lives as parents.

I constantly remind my patients that "a woman's body is God's masterpiece – it was His last creation before He rested on the seventh day." It can carry a pregnancy for nine months, sustain the pregnancy in-utero until birth, nurture life inside and outside the body, give birth to another human, sustain many more things, and overcome infertility setbacks.

This book can help nurses, and other clinicians in this field become more aware of the non-clinical and multifactorial layers of stressors that inevitably accompany an infertility diagnosis and affect the overall outcome of medical interventions. I found patients achieved a more successful result when the clinical team acknowledged and supported these private struggles.

The personal accounts of the patients in Part Two of this book reveal the dimensions of the inner core of the world of infertility. With a limited amount of resources available to tackle all the infertility difficulties, the patient often feels alone. Family and friends might provide only a small amount of support to help the patient deal with the stigma and shame of being "barren."

For some patients, their clinicians' expertise, transparency, and honesty help them navigate the intimidating maze in the world of infertility. Reducing their fear and stress helps them win this battle. They finally held their babies conceived by In-Vitro Fertilization (IVF). The routes to parenthood vary: using their own eggs (autologous), anonymous donor eggs, known-donor eggs, anonymous donor sperm, and anonymously donated embryos. Some turned to adoption when all else failed.

This book's accounts are for everyone globally who has been touched with a diagnosis of infertility and lived through the tornados of destruction it caused to their marriages, relationships, finances, friendships, self-esteem, self-worth, and faith. It is also for their relatives, friends, and clinicians who are there to offer meaningful support and guidance. The costs are high to fulfill the most natural biological instinct – motherhood and fatherhood.

Barren recounts women's journeys who also had to take a bold step to cross that abyss of anonymity and uncertainty. They embarked on their journey when they had no other choice but to use donor eggs, donor sperm, or donated embryos in pursuit of the longing to become parents. By doing so, they quelled the shame of infertility. Becoming a parent healed the jarring emotional, psychological, spiritual, and financial wounds they suffered for the privilege of blissfully changing their babies' diapers at midnight instead of the pangs of private sorrows of being barren.

Each woman's story is by no means pale compared to her fellow women's, but all suffered the same pain of stigma, hopelessness, isolation, relationship stress, spiritual, financial, and psychosocial dilemmas. Most but not all who achieved their dream of becoming a parent had a happy ending.

In Part Two of this book, the common denominators in the patient stories are their diagnosis, their determination to achieve success, and the infertility clinicians who held their hands and coached them through the rugged terrain of their journey to celebrate their victories ultimately. All these women, except one, were blessed to look at the faces of their babies who forever changed their lives.

No woman expects to face infertility, a path filled with shock, grief, stigma, despair, and uncertainties. But when it is the only avenue to fulfilling her most natural desire to become a mom, the bargaining chips are both the clinical diagnoses and the non-clinical factors *Barren* reveals. The path splits into two endpoints: a baby or empty arm.

As an infertility nurse for over a decade, I witnessed how this complex world resulted in brokenness and shame that shredded the fabric of women's self-worth, self-esteem, and men's egos and masculinity. I often see the lack of room for them to get their mind and emotions in a healthy balance. How they acknowledge and surmount the elements of this journey affects their experience and its outcome. Part Three offers nursing tips for those who may have to take this journey to parenthood.

I included several short memoirs of some infertility patients designed to share their stories so that others reading them may be encouraged. These new parents will take you down their roller-coaster trails to parenthood, which they never thought – even in their wildest dreams – to travel. You will understand some of the costly elements that added to their struggles.

For some of them, writing about their journey caused them to revisit a place they thought they left. Telling their stories served as therapy in putting more closure on that part of their lives. As you will come to understand, the world of infertility is often consumed by stress, blame, uncertainties, emotional breakdowns, and secrets, but in most cases produces the greatest love and purest joy in their babies' arrivals via birth and adoption.

This book sheds light on these women's unadulterated challenges outside of the normal scope of medical practice. Infertility facility staff typically focus on making a medical diagnosis and formulating a scientific biological treatment to cure infertility, but what about the patient's wholeness?

The couples featured in this book shared precious nuggets from their experiences that will help other women and their families to manage their expectations better when other non-clinical infertility struggles arise. I give much credit to science, technology, and cutting-edge procedures that were developed to overcome the many challenges, and to the infertility specialists, and their medical teams.

Also, the clinical staff has the power to look beyond the medical diagnoses to help identify the psychological and emotional signals of inner struggles so they can address and help overcome them. Just a kind word acknowledging a woman's private struggle can open a well of grief and shame, and offer some inner relief. One kind word can heal a profound wound.

From the perspective of some, infertility is worse than cancer. An infertility diagnosis not only dares to put an end to a woman's desires to be a mother and secure her posterity but forces her to painfully watch others around her fulfill that same desire without any challenges or setbacks. Infertile women see the headlines of abandoned babies or of babies being abused to death by parents, caregivers, and strangers. Why? How can this happen when others struggle to have a baby and embrace the purest form of bliss?

This book highlights infertile couples' struggles and triumphs and provides hope and inspiration for those who need to take this path.

Contents

Part One
The Medicine

Introduction	1
Chapter 1: Infertility Diagnoses	11
Chapter 2: Treatment Plans	35
Chapter 3: Pre-Implantation Genetic Testing	59
Chapter 4: Cost and Insurance Coverage	73
Chapter 5: Navigating the Multi-layer and Complicated Journey of Infertility	87
Chapter 6: The World of Infertility in the Pandemic	91

Part Two
It Happened to Me: Patients' Stories

Chapter 7: Margaret Davies	99
Chapter 8: Melissa and Josh Petrella	115
Chapter 9: Casandra and Daniel Williams	127
Chapter 10: Jill and Jack Hudson	133
Chapter 11: Sadie Blackwell	147
Chapter 12: Annabelle Theisen	179
Chapter 13: Prudence and Nate Smith	187
Chapter 14: Rochelle and Damian Henderson	193
Chapter 15: Nola and Brian Anderson	201
Chapter 16: Dustin and Caren Moore	209

Part Three
The Hidden Costs

Chapter 17: Relationships and Truths	215
Chapter 18: The Reality of Stigma, Grief, Shame, Fear, and Uncertainty	221

Chapter 19: Financial Implications 231
Chapter 20: God, Faith, and Religion 235
Chapter 21: Psychological, Moral, and Ethical Impacts 241
Chapter 22: Anonymity, Current DNA, and Genealogy Testing 251
Chapter 23: Fertility Preservation: The Non-Infertile Population 257
Chapter 24: Alternative Medicine and Its Impact on Pregnancy Outcomes 261
Chapter 25: Don't Go on this Journey Alone 271
Glossary 275
Citations 293
Consider Writing a Review 299

INTRODUCTION

In this book, I share with you the riveting stories of "hope almost lost" for women and couples who almost lost everything – their hope, faith, money, relationships, careers – for the goal of cradling a baby in their arms. Each woman's account brings the reality of stigma, loss, grief, decreased self-esteem, hopelessness, and second-guessing their spiritual, moral, and ethical beliefs that define the fabric of their existence. They felt despair their medical providers often did not recognize or effectively dealt with. The invisible despair resulted in them feeling more wounded and alone than they have ever imagined. *Barren* is story filled with these emotions.

Equally important, these stories also bring to light what the infertile couples overcame in reaching the gut-wrenching secretive decisions to use donor oocytes (another woman's eggs), donor sperm, and donated embryos to achieve parenthood at all cost.

"Barren" is a searing word for women and men who are having difficulties conceiving naturally. To those who have children without any problem, and those who do not care to have children, *barren* or infertile is just another word in the dictionary. As defined by the American Society of Reproductive Medicine (ASRM), infertility is the inability to conceive after 12 months (in women younger than 35 years old) of unprotected intercourse with a male partner or therapeutic donor sperm insemination, or 6 months in women older than 35 with a male partner or therapeutic donor sperm insemination (Infertility Work-up for The Women's Health Specialists, 2019).

Adding to the "duration" of failed attempts to conceive naturally, ASRM further describes infertility as the result of a disease (interruption, cessation, or disorder of the body function, systems, or organs) of the male or female reproductive tract. These factors prevent the conception of a child or the ability to carry a pregnancy to delivery (see Chapter 1).

According to the most recent data by the Centers for Disease Control and Prevention (CDC), 1 in every 7 American is impacted by the inability to conceive naturally. In other words, over 14 percent of the U.S. population of childbearing age is infertile – this includes both male and female (Reproductive Health, Infertility FAQs, n.d)

Both the CDC and SART (Society of Reproductive Technology) data reflect an increase in the volume of in-vitro fertilization (IVF) procedures since the 2008 economic downturn. Thus, the data has continued to rise astoundingly each year. At present, the data shows a 15% annual increase in seven out of the past eight years of Americans needing to turn to assisted reproductive technology (ART) procedures. The goal is to achieve pregnancy and build their families.

Introduction

But behind these data are the unmeasured non-medical prices the infertile woman or man pays: emotional, psychological, psychosocial, financial, moral, ethical, and spiritual.

- How do you measure a sense of loss, fear, relationship challenges, depletion of money, self-worth, self-esteem, faith, stigma, or pain inflicted emotionally and psychologically of being barren?

- How can you measure the elephant in the room – the strains in relationships, finances, faith, and the potential decline in overall productivity?

- How do you set a price on the consequences as women and couples grapple with the barriers and stigma of infertility, and the possibility of ending up childless for the rest of their lives, or their failure to produce a sibling for an only child?

I have worked in the field of infertility for more than a decade now and played an integral part of this multifactorial, stress-provoking journey of many women. Those who succeeded continue to keep me updated on their new journey as parents.

This book contains several infertility memoirs of women and couples who achieved parenthood through ART utilizing autologous (their own) egg, donor eggs, donor sperm, or a donated embryo. There are also the accounts of those who were not successful with ART procedures but are parents through the beautiful gift of adoption. Although the patients achieved parenthood because of perseverance and much more, there were many ups and downs. The patients navigated to challenges the best of their abilities, and often alone.

Barren highlights what the patients lived through and focuses on the clinicians and how they treated the patients. To most, it was about data, success ratings, and business as usual, but to a few, including nurses and others, infertility care is more than these factors. "Hilary Clinton said it takes a village to raise a child, but I say it takes a team to make one," says my co-worker, Sylvia Parrett, RN.

Infertility care includes strange stories:

- A husband who deliberately (or due to cold feet) did not show up to provide a sperm sample on the day of his wife's egg retrieval.

- An embryo that disappeared between thawing and final check under the microscope before the transfer procedure.

- The donor-egg recipient who attempted to hide among the waiting room of patients to get a glimpse of her anonymous egg donor on the day of her egg retrieval.

- The woman who attempted pregnancy by artificial insemination with her husband's sperm – with no infertility reason other than he was gay and still in the closet and not having sex with his wife.

It is not true that *only* older women turn to fertility treatment because of their ticking biological clocks. Many younger women and men, who never considered the possibility of being infertile, are shocked by such a diagnosis. While still reeling from the shock and grief, they must start

Introduction

the journey through the infertility world's maze. That first step may be intimidating, but it is essential.

The current generations focus on life's everyday challenges and efforts to shape their future with a college education, careers, financial stability, and other life endeavors. Consequently, they take preventative methods to avoid pregnancy at all costs until all they achieve other goals. Women especially take precautionary measures before marriage and even afterward only to find out later that there was no need. On the other hand, men use condoms or other methods to NOT impregnate a woman (and avoid sexually transmitted diseases). Unbeknownst to him, he was infertile all along. But then the time comes when the foundation of their lives is laid, and it is time to do what they ultimately want to do – procreate and build a family. They discover, to their surprise, they may be infertile.

As in the patriarchal times, infertility is still commonly focused on women primarily and, in many cases, women *only*. This myth dates to ancient times when a woman's only purpose was to take care of a man and make sure she produced his offspring. Thanks to the ever-evolving discoveries through science and technology, the naked truth comes out that "infertility," or "barrenness" is not only a female disease. It is equally a man's disease as well… so men are not removed from this equation any longer.

According to the U.S. Department of Health & Human Services (HHS), the Mayo Clinic, and the American Pregnancy Association (to name a few), "About one-third of infertility cases are caused by fertility problems in men, and another one-third of fertility problems are due to fertility problems in women. The other cases are caused by a mixture of male and female problems or by unknown problems". (How Common is Male Infertility and What are Its Causes? N.d). Infertility strikes men too. Male infertility is as real as female infertility, but more blame is placed on the female because she carries the pregnancy.

Couples who receive a diagnosis of infertility initially feel shocked and dismayed. Overcoming this challenge seems dismal, and women, men, and couples feel hit by a curveball before they can move to the question, "Is there a way to fix this problem?"

There are many ways to fix the issues. The solution depends on the diagnosis, the necessary procedures, the financial cost, and the prognosis. Other costs include emotional and psychological despair, cultural expectation, family, religious, and additional aspects of the stigma associated with this disease.

Dr. Connie Shapiro (2010) stated current research has shown that the stress levels of women with infertility are equivalent to women with cancer, AIDS, or heart disease, so there is no question about infertility resulting in enormous stress. Men also feel the pressure, and oftentimes perceive they are "less than a man" when the infertility tests pinpoint them.

Introduction

In patriarchal times, if a woman could not bear a child, her husband often discarded her for a new or additional wife. Now, with science and research information identifying the sources of both men and women, couples need to embrace the diagnosis without placing blame. The significant difference now only lies in the coping skills of men versus women and how they approach the journey of infertility treatments.

When a woman achieves her career goals but finds herself fallen short of her relationship goals, she has the option of freezing her eggs with the hope that she can find the man of her dreams eventually to fertilize those frozen eggs to have her babies. When this plan fails, many women find themselves going to the extreme of buying donated sperm to fertilize her banked frozen eggs to have her baby. Because she has the uterus to carry the fetus, and her body does the nurturing inside, she may conclude she does not need a man; she can buy sperm.

Almost all the infertility diagnoses lead to alternative methods of becoming a parent, whether by artificial insemination, the least invasive of infertility treatments, in-vitro fertilization (IVF) with the couple's eggs and sperm, IVF with donor eggs and/or donor sperm, or IVF with embryo donation and adoption. Becoming a parent is often dependent on how far a woman or a couple wants to go to become biological parents.

Part One

THE MEDICINE

Chapter 1

Infertility Diagnoses

The most recent data indicates that more than 7 million Americans are subject to an infertility diagnosis. Some do not classify infertility as a "disease" and may refer to this diagnosis as a reproductive abnormality, just a physical impairment, or a symptom of a male or female factor. Factoring age into the definition is pertinent and may be a symptom, given age is not a physical impairment but the natural process of life. However, the World Health Organization considers infertility a disease of the reproductive system irrespective of physical or clinical impairment and age.

A woman's eggs reserve (both quantity and quality) decreases with age. Studies prove a woman's fertility drops significantly after age 35, but the same is not true of a man. By revising the definition to include the impact of a woman's age, physicians can better encourage an earlier evaluation and treatment for their patients, which have proven to lead to more successful outcomes. As a result of this revised definition, women (and their male partners) become more aware of their fertility and proactively seek clinical evaluation and interventions earlier if they want to have children.

The woman's age factor may be more responsible for chromosomal abnormalities such as aneuploidy (a chromosomal mutation where there are too many or too few chromosomes). The sperm factor also negatively impacts pregnancy outcomes. One chromosome abnormality is Down's syndrome, also known as trisomy. There are three copies of chromosome 21 instead of the normal two copies in all cells. This extra copy results from an abnormal sperm cell (male) or egg cell (female) division in the development stage that would result in a chromosomal abnormality in the embryo.

The diagnostic phase of infertility is one of those "holding-your-breath-waiting-for-results" types of anxiety. This phase subjects the patients to many tests and procedures. The infertility diagnosis often results in shock for patients as they discover their inability to conceive was a result of a male or female diagnosis – or both, and in one-third of the cases – a diagnosis of unexplained infertility (an unknown factor).

Unexplained Infertility is both a male and a female diagnosis derived when there is no identified physical impairment. The impairments include blocked fallopian tubes or varicocele, insufficiencies such as low egg reserve or sperm count, or genetic disorder. Unexplained infertility can be associated with primary or secondary infertility. *Primary infertility* describes a woman who has never been pregnant before. *Secondary infertility* occurs when a previously pregnant woman delivered a baby and has difficulty achieving another pregnancy. Difficulties with sperm, eggs, tubes, or complications from prior pregnancy or surgery may cause secondary infertility.

Female Infertility Diagnoses encompass many factors; egg reserve (quantity of eggs) and egg quality are on top of the list. Other causes include advanced reproductive age (ARA equal or greater than 36 years), blocked fallopian tubes (often caused by ectopic pregnancy, salpinges, cysts, endometriosis, or sexually transmitted diseases), ovulation disorder, polycystic ovarian syndrome (**PCOS**), unhealthy body weights, thyroid issues, uterine factors, history of pelvic inflammatory diseases (**PID**) often caused by sexually transmitted infections such as gonorrhea and chlamydia, cancer treatment, and genetic disorders.

Advanced Reproductive Age (ARA) affects a woman as she ages. Not only does her egg count diminishes, but also the quality. Poor egg quality leads to abnormal fertilization. ARA impacts the integrity and ability of a woman's eggs to be fertilized. Many miscarriages are related to abnormal fertilization due to chromosomal issues, as mentioned earlier.

Diminished Ovarian Reserve (DOR) occurs when a woman's egg (oocytes) count and egg quality significantly decreased. This happens when a woman's ovaries lose their potential to produce and mature their eggs. DOR typically occurs as a woman ages but also afflicts younger women as well. When ovarian reserve drastically declines in younger women, the diagnosis is termed "premature ovarian failure or insufficiency– POF or POI".

A woman is born with all the eggs she will ever have, and over time the DNA changes and the eggs degenerate, resulting in poor quality. The most rapid degeneration occurs between 10-15 years *before* menopause. Unlike men, who have a continuous formation of sperm cells with full maturation over 3-4 months, women are born with eggs that develop by the twenty-fourth week of gestation, making them among the longest-lived cells in the body. By the end of the second trimester (around the twenty-fourth week of pregnancy) a female fetus has 7-20 million oocytes, with this number decreasing to 1-2 million by birth, 400,000 by puberty, and finally drops to less than 10,000 by menopause. Although an egg or two achieve full maturation during the menstrual cycle, a "crop" (many) eggs get released each month, and as a woman ages, that crop becomes smaller.

- Unlike men, the quality of a woman's eggs is impacted negatively by age. The rate at which the egg reserve and quality decrease is affected by age primarily. Lifestyle habits such as smoking tobacco and certain foods also affect egg quality.
- A few stories in this book, such as Casandra's (Chapter 9) and Sadie's (Chapter 11) provide first-hand accounts of women who had their babies by egg and embryo donation because of DOR and POF/POI.
- Although these are real infertility issues, some women are in denial and do not understand the reality and real implications of the inability to conceive with their own eggs.

Female Hormones

- A simple blood test to measure Anti-Mullerian Hormone (AMH) and Follicular Stimulating Hormone (FSH) give an indicator of diminished ovarian levels. As the AMH decreases to below 1.0 ng/ml and the FSH rises above 10.0 IU/ml, a woman's egg reserve also diminishes, reducing the chances of becoming pregnant. With age, the quality of the human egg degenerates, as mentioned above. The egg quality inhibits its ability to fertilize normally to become a viable pregnancy decreases and leads to a negative pregnancy test result after a conception attempt or early miscarriages.

- When female hormones become abnormal, in-vitro fertilization (IVF) provides solutions. Donor eggs may be the best option for having a baby when there is a significantly decreased or undetectable egg supply or quality.

The average normal range of AMH in women of child-bearing age is 1.0 – 4.0 ng/ml, and FSH is less than 15 I.U./ml on day 3 of menses. (FSH level changes from month to month – and between days 2-5 of menses). Healthcare providers are concerned when the day 3 level is consistently above 10, but more concerned when it is closer to 15. So, technically a consistent increase between 10-15 sends a red flag the egg reserve is on the decline.

To comprehend the clinical implications of an elevated FSH and decreased AMH in women who want to have a baby with their own eggs, physicians must understand why these hormone levels increase and decrease. An ultrasound that measures the antra-follicle count (AFC) between days 2-5 often correlates to the egg reserve.

FSH is a follicular stimulating hormone released by the pituitary gland in the brain. In the beginning of a menstrual period, this level tends to be on the lower end of normal (normal is about 4-15) in women of childbearing age. This hormone's level indicates the amount of stimulation the brain needs to mature follicles (eggs).

This level increases during the eggs' maturation phase and therefore rises every day of the maturation phase (days 1-14 of menses). The FSH level *peaks* before ovulation, signaling the ovary to release the mature egg(s). When that egg is released, the FSH level dips.

Measuring the FSH level near day 3 of a menstrual cycle indicates eggs reserve. When that egg reserve is *low*, the brain works harder to stimulate FSH levels, causing FSH to *rise higher than normal*.

AMH is a hormone that indicates the amount of eggs a woman has; hence physicians use this level to estimate egg count. This level usually correlates to the antra-follicle count (AFC), the number of potential eggs seen on the ultrasound on days 2-3 of a menstrual cycle. So, when there is a *low* AMH, there is also a *low* number of antra-follicles.

The AMH level indicates egg reserve but in the *opposite* way as FSH, when AMH is lower than 1.0 ng/ml (normal range - 1.0–4.0 ng/ml). FSH is typically higher than normal on days 2-3 of a menstrual cycle.

- As mentioned earlier, quite a few factors impact a woman's fertility. Clinically, doctors use three tests to measure a woman's ovarian reserve: AMH, FSH, and AFC (antra-follicle count done by ultrasound). Below is a chart to help you understand these levels. FSH and AFC are typically measured on days 2-3 of menses. AMH can be measured at any time of the month as it is more constant.

- Note: As age increases, FSH increases. But as FSH increases, AMH and AFC decrease.

Laboratory Data: A pilot study done on IVF patients in collaboration with a group of three gynecologists — 105 samples for validating AMH ranges used for stratifying female infertile patients and diagnostic cut off correlating with PCOS.

Correlation of AMH levels for stratifying patients for IVF protocol and outcomes							
Age group	AMH Values (ng/ml)						FSH values (mIU/ml)
	Optimal	Satisfactory	Low fertility			Very low	High	Ave.
	4.0-6.79	2.19-4.0	0.3-1.0	1.0-1.5	1.5-2.19	<0.3	>6.79	
21-25 (8)	4	3	0	0	0	0	1	4.57
25-40 (89)	18	25	13	1	10	7	15	7.92
Above 40 (8)	0	0	0	0	0	8	0	20.34
IVF, pregnancy outcome							
	10 of 22 (44%)	12 of 28 (40%)	8 of 24 (33%)			4 of 15 (26%	3 of 16 (18%	
			2 of 13	1 of 1	5 of 10			

Slide Share (link: https://images.app.goo.gl/HGBpQLhBUPQ924yh7)

Sandra's Situation

Recently I encountered a 52-year-old woman in menopause (I will call her Sandra) who was adamant about getting insurance approval for IVF treatment using her own eggs. Considering Sandra's advanced reproductive age, her healthcare providers determined she had significantly diminished ovarian reserve. These factors were working against her:

- Advanced age

- An undetectable AMH (anti-Mullerian hormone) of less than 0.003 ng/ml (less than 1.0 ng/ml is a problem)

- Elevated FSH (follicular stimulating hormone) of 58 I.U./ml (higher than 10 I.U./ml is a problem)

- Despite my lengthy explanations, Sandra threatened to sue her insurance carrier if she was denied a prior-authorization approval for IVF using her own eggs. Sandra asserted her celebrity idol, Janet Jackson, had recently had a baby, so Sandra genuinely believed that she could as well. Sandra clearly had run out of eggs.

- Abnormal levels are mostly indicated in older women but are not uncommon in younger women, typically those with premature ovarian failure (POF). And although pregnancy is less than likely to occur naturally and easily for women with borderline low levels, it is possible. But it is almost impossible to conceive with autologous eggs (your own eggs) with extremely low or abnormal levels described above.

Ovarian Factors

Premature Ovarian Failure (POF), also referred to as premature ovarian insufficiency (POI), occurs in the younger population who is not expected to run out of eggs or go through menopause before turning forty. Unfortunately for some women, their ovaries stop functioning before 40 years of age. This is rare. The occurrence is one in 1,000 women under the age of 30 and one in 100 women under 40. The average onset is age 27 years (POF. Resolve.org). The initial symptoms are usually menstrual disorder, shortened and irregular periods.

Annabelle, who adopted two embryos and delivered healthy twin girls two years ago, found out about her POF diagnosis when she visited her gynecologist because of sporadic periods. She attributed this occurrence to a hectic professional lifestyle and frequent travel and was shocked to learn of her POF.

Polycystic Ovarian Syndrome is also a common hormonal disorder in women of reproductive age (21 years old-44 years old). This diagnosis is also characterized by irregular periods due to a high level of *male* hormones. Male hormones prevent the normal maturation of female eggs contributing to infertility in women. The words "poly" means "many or numerous," and "cystic" as in cysts gives rise to "polycystic" or many cysts (on the ovaries). These cysts are pockets of fluids formed on the periphery of the ovaries – they may each contain an immature egg that cannot come to full maturation or be released in a normal hormonal environment. Depending on the woman's age, PCOS is often measured by an AMH of greater than 5.0 ng/ml – this level can be even higher in much younger women. (AMH is high in PCOS – "polycystic ovarian syndrome). Women with PCOS also tend to be obese, have acne, excess hair growth, and have insulin resistance.

Ovulation Disorder (OD) is often associated with polycystic ovarian syndrome (PCOS), premature ovarian failure (POF), age-related diminished ovarian reserve (DOR), obesity impacting metabolism, irregular menstrual cycles, and hormonal imbalance.

Tubal Factors

Tubal Disease (tubal factor) is another common female infertility diagnosis. It affects 1 in 50 pregnancies (Ectopic Pregnancy, American Pregnancy Association). The fallopian tubes are the tunnels through which eggs travel downwards after they are released by the ovaries to meet the sperm cells that make their way upwards after intercourse or artificial insemination.

If there are blockages in these tubes, then the sperm cannot meet the eggs, and hence fertilization does not have a chance. There must be a "meet, greet, and fertilize process" between a normal sperm and a normal egg for a chance at fertilization. There are times when a sperm may find its way around to meet and fertilize an egg. But sometimes, in the early stage of this process, as the combined clump of cells divide and multiply, the pregnancy (zygote) gets stuck in one of the fallopian tubes resulting in an *ectopic* pregnancy. An ectopic pregnancy will not survive because it needs the nourishment and space in the uterus. The fallopian tube is only 4-5 inches long and 0.2 to 0.6 inches wide.

In a worst-case scenario, an ectopic pregnancy threatens the life of the woman when the tube ruptures and internal bleeding occurs. In many cases, the loss of a fallopian tube is inevitable with an ectopic (tubal) pregnancy. A surgeon must remove the ruptured tube. The loss of a tube decreases the chance to conceive by fifty percent.

Endometriosis and sexually transmitted diseases such as chlamydia result in tube scarring and are common causes for blockage within the fallopian tubes. Hydrosalpinx (also referred to as cyst) in the fallopian tube obstructs the passageway. Cysts may need to be surgically removed, resulting in the potential loss of use of tubes.

Bilateral tubal ligation (BTL) is a voluntary sterilization procedure that cuts or ties the fallopian tubes to prevent pregnancy for those who do not want to have children. This is not a disease but becomes a tubal factor if someone changes her mind after the procedure. An example is when a woman thought she didn't want more children but then, later on, finds herself in a new relationship with a partner who wants kids. In that case, she might undergo a sterilization reversal procedure. There is no guarantee that a reversal would be successful, and when unsuccessful, IVF is required.

Vardhini's Situation

Vardhini and Ramesh delayed having children until they reached a stable situation in their jobs. They owned a house and had well-paying jobs. Vardhini planned to return to her job after having their first child. In July, Vardhini found out she was pregnant. Shortly afterward, she developed sharp, stabbing abdominal pain, vaginal bleeding, and nausea. In the emergency department, after the ultrasound showed her uterus was empty, Vardhini and Ramesh learned Vardhini had an ectopic pregnancy. She underwent surgery to remove the ruptured tube and stop the bleeding.

Ramesh and Vardhini believed she could become pregnant as she had one tube left. One year later, Vardhini experienced the same symptoms shortly after she learned she was again pregnant. Heartbroken, she underwent a second surgery to save her life from the internal bleeding and remove the second ruptured fallopian tube.

After Vardhini recovered, the couple had a chance to seek counseling about their options. With the loss of both fallopian tubes, fertilization was only possible outside the body. Vardhini underwent IVF using her own eggs and her husband's sperm. The procedure worked the first time. Vardhini had some complications during her pregnancy, which required her to remain on bed rest for most of it. She delivered healthy twin girls, and the couple decided their family was complete.

Uterine Factors

Uterine disorder is commonly caused by:

- fibroids (non-cancerous tumors),
- septums (walls within the uterus),
- congenital abnormalities,
- cancer,
- endometritis (inflammation of the endometrium/wall of the uterus),
- scar tissues which can be associated with endometriosis,
- retained product of conception (**POC**) from a prior miscarriage and
- surgeries related to them.

Endometriosis is a medical condition in which the endometrium (lining inside the uterus/womb) grows outside of the uterus and attaches to surrounding organs such as ovaries, tubes, the bowel, and bladder. The cause of this disease is unknown, but researchers have a few theories – yet to be proven. This condition can be mild to severe and often quite painful.

In severe cases, a surgical procedure such as laparoscopy with ablations or removal of adhesions (bands of scar tissue) is done to remove the tissue. This process may scar the ovarian tissues and fallopian tube. While endometriosis can be decreased via this procedure, a couple of risks are a decrease in the ovarian reserve and the scarring or loss of a tube. These events decrease the chances of pregnancy.

Endometriosis is more common in the younger population. According to statistics, about five million women in America suffer from endometriosis, and according to the National Institute of Child and Human Developments, this number may be much higher for the mere fact that not everyone with endometriosis experience severe symptoms (Shriver, 2020).

Recurrent Pregnancy Loss is marked by two or more clinical pregnancy losses *before* 20 weeks of gestation. A clinical pregnancy is evidenced by high levels of hCG (the pregnancy hormone) and ultrasound confirmation of a gestational sac or fetal heartbeat. Detecting a fetal heartbeat with a handheld Doppler or a fetoscope also clinically confirms a pregnancy.

A clinical pregnancy does not include ectopic or biochemical pregnancies – these are defined and managed differently. Given that the definition of clinical pregnancy as a loss after a gestational sac within the uterus or a fetal heartbeat is detected, one cannot say that ectopic (tubal) or biochemical pregnancies are classified as RPL because a gestational sac or fetal heartbeat is not detected in these pregnancies.

This is because a biochemical occurs early (before 6 weeks) before a heartbeat can be detected on ultrasound, and a tubal pregnancy is not within the uterus but the tube(s).

A biochemical pregnancy does not get to the ultrasound confirmation stage - it is usually detected by a urine pregnancy test and sometimes a blood test. This hormone level rises and then drops to negative level followed by menses.

An ectopic (tubal) pregnancy is usually confirmed by the pattern of blood beta hCG levels. It rises appropriately, but then plateaus by the 6th week. The mother may feel pain; an ultrasound may or may not confirms the pregnancy.

Recurrent pregnancy loss is often referred to as *habitual abortion*. Approximately 15% of all clinical pregnancies fail before twenty weeks of gestation, and roughly 1-2 percent of these women experience recurrent or habitual losses.

Generally, a miscarriage, known as a spontaneous abortion (SAB), recurrent or not, can be in the form of sudden bleeding and passing the product of conception (POC) or the absence of fetal heartbeat detected by ultrasound. These may be managed and treated differently, either by monitoring the pregnancy hormone (beta hCG) levels until it goes to zero or by dilatation and curettage (D&C) with frequent monitoring of the beta hCG level to zero.

This diagnosis can be in a league of its own. Although RPL is not truly labeled as an infertility diagnosis, women are referred to a reproductive endocrinologist (infertility specialist) for a workup to identify the cause and determine a treatment plan to reduce the risk of further miscarriages. In cases of **RPL**, there is usually no hindrance in getting pregnant, but rather in *sustaining* the pregnancy. An autoimmune or genetic disorder may also be responsible for **RPL**.

Each pregnancy loss may be due to a different cause and must be studied individually. A woman may lose a child for several reasons, such as

- a result of a chromosomal abnormality, in which case **IVF** with pre-implantation genetic screening (**PGS**) can be performed to rule out genetically abnormal embryos (age related - older eggs) or genetic mutations, which leads to early miscarriages
- incompetent cervix (unable to stay closed for the duration of the pregnancy),
- infection within the uterus,
- untreated hypothyroidism,
- endocrine abnormalities,
- uncontrolled diabetes,
- uterine anatomic abnormalities,
- thrombophilia,
- antiphospholipid antibody syndrome (**APLS**), which is the presence of abnormal antibodies in the blood associated with abnormal blood clotting,
- protein insufficiency, and

- autosomal disorder where the body develops a rejection for embryonic cells.

When the etiology (origin of disease) is known, then treatment can be determined. Therefore, the physician must investigate the cause of a patient's RPL because defining the reason and requiring diagnostic testing and therapeutic intervention rests on the clinician's knowledge and expertise to reduce the risk for subsequent fetal loss. Once the cause is identified and treated, a woman can go on to become pregnant again and be able to sustain the pregnancy to delivery.

Although a spontaneous pregnancy loss is both physically and emotionally taxing for couples, these feelings of grief, despair, and uncertainty for future pregnancy success can be exponential, especially when faced with recurrent losses.

When celebrities are vocal about their struggle, it removes some of the stigma, and others become less reluctant to be open about their losses and seek professional care.

The Duchess of Sussex, Megan Markle, spoke about the feelings of grief she and her husband Prince Harry experienced with the miscarriage of their second child in 2020. Megan said, "Losing a child means carrying an almost unbearable grief, experienced by many but talked about by few, and despite the staggering commonality of this pain, the conversation remains taboo, riddled with (unwarranted) shame, and perpetuating a cycle of solitary mourning" (Picheta, 2020).

Social media followed two celebrities who opened up about the unimaginable grief and sadness of their pregnancy losses. Yoga instructor and wife of Alec Baldwin, Hilaria suffered two miscarriages – one at 20 weeks and after another loss a few months before. The other celebrity is cookbook author and wife of John Legend, Chrissy Teigen, who wrote an essay about losing her son, Jack, at 20 weeks to the diagnosis of "partial placenta abruption,"

According to the American College of Obstetrics and Gynecologists, around 10% of all pregnancies end in miscarriages (FAQs. Early Pregnancy Loss). However, health care in America has not mastered the art and science of implementing adequate interventions to heal the broken spirit and emotional hurt these women face. Interventions to help make sense and bring healing in all these categories is needful.

The infertility world typically focuses on women with a RPL diagnosis in finding the cause and treatment, but effective emotional and psychological interventions can miss the mark. In rare cases, a fertility specialist offers a social worker or behavioral psychologist; many patients and their significant other are not ready to take the offer. Often, the blame game takes preeminence; either the female blames herself or her partner.

Many couples face much loss and grief when an unexpected miscarriage occurs, and the suffering can be multiplied when pregnancy first needed to be achieved via IVF or FET.

Other Factors

Autoimmune Disorder: Although this factor may not be a common infertility diagnosis, for those who are diagnosed, the road to achieving a baby can become even more tedious and tiring. There are a host of auto-immunologic diseases that affect infertility in both men and women. They include celiac disease, lupus, and hypothyroidism in women. Men may have an autoimmune mechanism to induce high anti-seminal/sperm antibodies that work against fertilization. When these are not detected, it could account for a portion of "unexplained infertility." One of the reasons is because autoimmune disorders – which are rare – leading to infertility may be understudied, and there are not very many experts in the field.

As you will read in Part Two, one of my patients was diagnosed with Sjögren's syndrome – an autoimmune disease that hampered her attempts to conceive. As high as 4.8% of the general population is diagnosed with this autoimmune disorder, and according to Suruchi Gupta and Nikhil Gupta, "Women with Sjögren syndrome require prenatal counseling explaining the risks involved and the need to control the disease well before conception" (Gupta, 2017).

This disorder affects the connective tissues, making conception and pregnancy more difficult. Women suffering from this condition usually have antibodies known as *antiphospholipid*, which makes the blood more prone to clotting. As a result, miscarriages are more likely to occur because the placenta's blood can clot easily.

Radiation and chemotherapy can inevitably render both female and male infertile. Exposure to radiation and cancer treatment drugs such as chemotherapy and surgery reduces fertility. Radiation is not good for a fetus. Therefore, healthcare providers ask women about the possibility of being pregnant at the time of x-rays and are provided with a shield against radiation.

Chemotherapy works as a cancer treatment in killing off both cancer cells and healthy cells. Eggs and sperms are affected by these treatments. Therefore, patients in child-bearing years have the choice of undergoing procedures to preserve eggs and freeze sperm before starting cancer treatment if possible. Children conceived from cryopreserved (frozen) egg and sperm cells before cancer treatment are not at risk of having cancer as a result.

Cancer surgeries, depending on the type, can also lead to infertility. Two types of cancer-related surgeries in women are removing ovaries (oophorectomy) and the uterus (hysterectomy). Removal of the testes can render a male infertile.

Male Infertility

According to the American Society of Reproductive Medicine (ASRM), 10-15% of couples in the United States are infertile. About one percent of men in the total global and U.S. population are diagnosed with azoospermia (no sperm). There is a 40-50% percent of infertility cases linked to a male factor globally.

Semen Analysis

The first step in diagnosing a male contribution to infertility is a semen analysis. Common issues surround four parameters of a semen analysis: volume, concentration/count, motility, and morphology. The normal volume of sperm in one ejaculate is approximately 1.5 milliliters (ml). There should be at least 15 million sperm per ml (the concentration), bringing the total to approximately 25 million sperm per ejaculate (the count).

- The other two parameters that define the health of an ejaculate are normal motility percentage *greater than 40*. In contrast, the normal percentage of morphology (shape) is greater than 4% on a Kruger criterion (standardized scale) in fertile men ages 20 - 50 years old.

- Male infertility is more common than you think, and the most common diagnosis is azoospermia or no sperm. Other factors can stem from low sperm count, low motility, or abnormal morphology (shape) of sperm.

- Azoospermia (no sperm) or a decreased sperm production may be mechanical due to an obstructive (15% of cases) or a non-obstructive (85% of cases) issue. The "unexplained" azoospermia is due to a micro-deletion of the Y (male) chromosomes, failure to fully mature the sperm, or abnormal chromosomes analysis in number or appearance.

Other contributing male factors are
- undescended testicles,
- varicocele (enlarged veins in the testes),

- genetic disorder,
- infections such as HIV, gonorrhea, and chlamydia, and
- diabetes.

According to the American Pregnancy Association (Male Infertility, 2018) there are four main causes of male infertility, and below is a percentage of distribution:

- Hypothalamic or pituitary disorder (1-2%)
- Gonad (testicles) disorder (30-40%)
- Sperm transport disorder (10-20%)
- Unknown causes (40-50%)

There are a few techniques that can be used to increase the effectiveness of sperm to cause pregnancy. A semen analysis is vital in determining the sperm's ability to fertilize an egg and helps the provider decide if specialized techniques need to increase the fertilization rate.

a. **Intracytoplasmic sperm injection (ICSI)** versus insemination are procedures determined primarily by the semen analysis' four measured parameters.

b. **The ZyMot Device**: The Zyot Device is an FDA-approved device currently on the market. Some clinics are now using it to isolate the healthiest, best-performing sperm for IUI, (Intrauterine Insemination) IVF, and ICSI. (The ZyMot Multi (380) sperm separation device, n.d.)

c. **Sperm Cap-Score Assay** is a recent groundbreaking technology believed to be a major determinant of whether the sperm can fertilize an egg.

(The Cap-Score Sperm Function Test is a laboratory-developed test which is not available in many countries but is available in the United States.) A poor Cap-Score is an indicator of the sperm's limited ability to penetrate and fertilize an egg.

Cap refers to capacitation or the process the sperm goes through to fertilize an egg successfully. The test measures its ability to start an appropriate swimming pattern through the cervix, into the fallopian tube, and through the egg's outer cover. This journey of the sperm must reckon with the effects of the female reproductive tract. As the sperm makes this journey, enzymes are released that enables it to pass between cells surrounding and protect the egg's outer covering.

Paul and Erica's Situation

Female eggs can be picky and reject partner's sperm. On the other hand, semen can cause an immune response in his body or his partner's body. That immune response results in the formation of antibodies that can damage or kill the sperm cells, ultimately making it difficult for fertilization. There must be compatibility of receptors between the eggs and the sperm to achieve fertilization.

Paul and Erica could not conceive in over ten years of marriage. They loved each other very much but divorced due to the stressors of not having children. Their case was a rare one. There was a clinical incompatibility with their sperm and egg. Though limited, studies have indicated that there are potentially incompatible receptors of both the eggs and the sperm for conception to take place. Though they each had no clinical barrier, they failed to become pregnant without and with treatment. Their diagnosis was "unexplained" infertility. Although it is not a true allergy, some non-medical people refer to this as being allergic to each other's eggs and sperm.

After Paul's infidelity led to impregnating another woman, their marriage ended. Erica quickly became pregnant with her new husband and completed her family with two daughters and a son.

After several years and teenage kids, Erica and Paul came to terms with the end of their marriage and knew they failed because of unexplained infertility as a couple. Now with the Sperm Cap-Score test and the ZyMot procedure, couples may be able to overcome such heartbreaks.

Obstructive issues also affect male fertility. Varicocele is an enlargement in a vein within the scrotum that can result in low sperm production and decreased sperm quality. This is usually common in younger men but can be present in older men and can cause no symptoms. Physicians can overcome blockages that result from varicocele and hinder conception by a testicular biopsy procedure known as Testicular Sperm Extraction (TESE), typically done by a urologist. Factors contributing to this male factor are undescended testicles (mostly diagnosed in infants), absence of vas deferens (the tube that carries sperm from the testicle to the penis), and genetic disorders, such as cystic fibrosis.

Chapter 2

Treatment Plans

History of Donations

It is likely that in 1953, the first baby from a sperm donation was born. The procedure for sperm donation has not changed much since then except for strict FDA regulations and more careful screening of the sperm donors to rule out diseases.

The advances of infertility medicine have come an exceptionally long way since the first IVF success in 1978. Born to British parents, Louise Brown, now 42 years old, was the first "test tube baby" in the world.

The first donor egg baby happened six years later in 1984; the procedure was quite different than today. The donor received sperm from the recipient's husband through artificial insemination. The physician transferred the fertilized egg (embryo) after it began to develop from the donor's uterus in whom it had been conceived to the woman who gave birth to the full-term infant. This procedure is outdated. In the current procedure, the eggs are harvested from the donor, fertilized in the lab, and transferred from the petri dish (test tube) to the recipient's uterus.

Embryo donation is the newer form of advanced reproductive technology, and no one really knows of the first baby born from a donated embryo.

Less Invasive Treatment Choices

An infertile couple faces options for treatment. After the initial shock of hearing the diagnosis of infertility, the couple often wants to know what they can do to help them achieve their goal of having a baby. In response, healthcare providers first offer the most common treatment options, which are less invasive (not as complicated). There are more aggressive therapies if the first line of treatment does not work after a few cycles. The providers might also suggest more aggressive treatment for blocked or missing fallopian tubes, low egg, low sperm counts, and genetic disorders.

Less invasive treatment plans are a starting point for couples who have been trying on their own to achieve pregnancy but failed. These plans include Timed-Intercourse (TIC) with or without medications or intrauterine inseminations (IUI) with or without medications depending on their clinical history.

Timed intercourse without medications

Suppose Henrietta has adequate eggs reserve, patent fallopian tubes, and a somewhat predictable ovulation. Her male partner does not have a male factor. Timed intercourse (TIC) cycle would be the first line of treatment. Closer monitoring with blood tests and ultrasound to determine the optimal window for conception is the most that may be done at this point. This is a typical case of unexplained infertility where there is no identifiable hindrance regarding the sperm and egg meeting.

Timed intercourse with medications

Suppose Juanita has irregular ovulation. She may need to take Clomid or Letrozole tablets for about five days to help make ovulation predictable. Pregnancy may result from being able to manipulate the ovulation timing. These medications are also used in a woman who ovulates regularly but still has difficulty conceiving because she is not recruiting (creating an egg or two that goes into the fallopian tube) per cycle. Clomid or Letrozole results in producing more than *one egg* per cycle, which increases the probability of pregnancy. The success rate is 10-20% per cycle. The risk of having twins is about 8-10%, and the risk of having triplets is about 1% (Multiple Pregnancy and Birth: Twins, Triplets, and High Order Multiples, ASRM).

Clomid, Letrozole, and low dose injectable medications treat predictable ovulations but lower the egg numbers when the goal is to stimulate the ovaries to recruit more than one egg but less than three. A trigger shot like Ovidrel may be part of these types of treatment plans. Letrozole is more effective in women with polycystic ovarian syndrome (PCOS).

Intrauterine inseminations (IUI) without medication

Healthcare providers refer to an unmedicated IUI cycle, also referred to as a "natural cycle." It is "natural" and does not require medication to stimulate the development of a follicle because the woman's body does that independently. Typically, an unmedicated cycle is the line of treatment for women who have a good egg reserve and predictable ovulation, as mentioned in Henrietta's case. Still, there is a male factor such as an abnormal semen analysis. Although medication is not needed to induce egg recruitment, heterosexual couples with a male factor diagnosis, single women using donor sperm, or same-sex female using donor sperm, the IUI procedure is needed. A trigger injection such as Ovidrel may stimulate the mature egg's release from the ovary into the fallopian tube to meet the sperm at a predicted time. Even though a trigger injection may be unnecessary, it enhances the process.

Intrauterine inseminations (IUI) with medication

A medicated IUI cycle requires the use of follicular stimulating or ovulation-inducing drugs. The follicular stimulating drugs help recruit 1-3 eggs minimum per month to optimize at least one fertilizer probability. This occurs when there is a normal egg reserve, but the body does not mature the eggs by ovulation, or the ovulation window is unpredictable. The woman receives Clomid, Letrozole and some injectable medications such as Gonal-f, Follistim, and Menopur (FSH injectable medications). These medications regulate ovulation in cases when ovulation is not predictable, such as in women with irregular menstrual cycles, ovulation disorder, and PCOS, and also recruit a few eggs. In cases of normal semen analysis, TIC may be encouraged, but if there is a male factor as well, IUI will give a better outcome.

With an IUI treatment plan, all the lab-prepared viable sperm in concentrated form are placed directly into the uterus via a very thin catheter, eliminating the sperm's loss outside the uterus. A sperm-wash (sperm preparation) is performed in the andrology lab at the clinic to enhance this process. The sperm wash also eliminates non-motile sperm before the insemination process.

A male semen sample comprises of sperm that are alive and dead. Sperm live for about 72 hours. The semen sample also contains mucus, enzymes, proteins, and fluid that are non-desirable in mixing with eggs to achieve fertilization. The sperm-washing process removes these extraneous particles. There are a few steps in preparing the sperm.

- **Warming**: Once the sample is collected, the andrologist places it in a warmer for 20 minutes to liquify.

- **Basic Analysis**: The andrologist runs a basic analysis of the sperm count, motility percentage, forward progression, volume, and viscosity.

- **Filter**: A gradient solution with different densities is added to the sample to act as a filter. Also added are antibiotics and protein supplements.

- **Centrifuge**: The semen sample is placed into a tube and the centrifuge where it spins on high speed allowing separation of the best sperm from debris and non-moving sperm.

- **Ready for Use:** The concentrated volume of the centrifuged sample is removed and added to a nourishing and preserving fluid called Human Tubal Fluid (HTF). The prepared sample is now ready for the insemination procedure.

Intrauterine insemination versus timed intercourse

A common question that women and couples ask is, "Why do we need to start TIC or IUI (medicated or unmedicated) treatment plan instead of just having sex?" A woman may attempt TIC and/or IUI during her workup's diagnostic phase while definitive tests such as a fallopian/uterine cavity study, hysterosalpingogram (HSG), semen analysis, and egg reserve test are in progress. Starting a TIC or IUI does not waste time because trying these treatment options may result in success.

Timed intercourse (TIC) is a simple treatment option for infertility. It involves monitoring a woman's ovulation cycle via ultrasound and hormone testing to detect the appropriate window to have intercourse to become pregnant. Having sexual intercourse around the time the woman is most fertile increases the chance of pregnancy. This is the first line of treatment for heterosexual couples who do not have anatomical or sperm and egg issues but need help predicting when is the optimal window in the menstrual cycle to become pregnant.

An intrauterine insemination (IUI) is an artificial insemination procedure, a deliberate introduction of sperm into a female's cervix or uterine cavity using a syringe (containing) attached a plastic tip at the appropriate ovulation time to achieve a pregnancy other than by sexual intercourse. Providers use this technique to ensure the concentrated amount of sperm produced is placed in the uterus at the appropriate time of ovulation. The sperm sample is washed and prepped before insemination. See "sperm washing" in the earlier paragraph.

Aggressive Treatment

Generally, health insurance plans provide infertility coverage for in-vitro fertilization (IVF) after the woman or couple demonstrates they have tried and failed these less aggressive (or less invasive) treatments before the plans approve IVF coverage.

Aggressive treatment plans such as IVF are recommended if the less invasive treatment plans fail to achieve pregnancy. IVF is medically necessary when couples failed several IUI cycles or there is evidence of a diminished ovarian reserve, blocked fallopian tube, missing fallopian tube(s), endometriosis, abnormal semen analysis, or known genetic disorder.

People used to label in-vitro fertilization as "test-tube pregnancy." It is the process of fertilizing the eggs with the sperm outside the woman's body. In the case of eggs, sperm, tubal, or genetic issues, this procedure is the most common approach to creating an embryo. However, many couples view it as shameful or abnormal and do not want others to know they chose this path. It is even more hidden when the woman or couple receives donor eggs and/or donor sperm to achieve parenthood.

One of the reasons why IVF is still a well-kept secret is because people do not want to expose themselves to the stigma of infertility. For some, this may no longer be as shameful because many celebrities have credited the IVF process to becoming parents. So, thanks to publicity, many celebrities are now discussing their experiences, and some infertile couples are less uncomfortable and a bit more open about this diagnosis.

Country singer Chuck Wicks learned his low sperm count was why his wife could not get pregnant during months of trying. The medical team used a stimulant on a fresh specimen of semen and located *two* sperm that were alive. Using two of his wife Kasi's eggs, the team injected each with a single sperm. One of the eggs was successfully fertilized. The embryo was frozen to be transferred two months later to Kasi's uterus. She needed to take hormone shots to prepare her uterus to accept the embryo and her body for the pregnancy. Genetic testing determined the embryo was healthy and would be a boy. The couple rejoiced in the success of the transplanted embryo (Kruh, 2020).

More aggressive plans might involve the use of donor eggs and donor embryos. This ART plan is still shrouded in secrecy. IVF with donor eggs is recommended for women who cannot produce adequate quantity and quality of eggs as evidenced by test results and/or failed attempts with their own eggs. This approach is a standard recommendation for advanced reproductive age, diminished ovarian reserve, and premature ovarian failure. In-vitro fertilization babies from egg or embryo donation are however, still an extremely well-kept secret.

There are women in their late 40s and early 50s (and as old as in their 60s) who have given birth to babies. Many in the general population believe these mothers used their own eggs. However, most of them used egg or embryo donors. These women are not likely to use their own cryopreserved (frozen) eggs from when they were in their 20s and 30s because fertility preservation treatments were very uncommon and using thawed eggs still does not have a great success rate.

Egg Donations and How They Work

Women diagnosed with diminished ovarian reserve, premature ovarian failure, endometriosis, or have had their ovaries removed need to use someone else's eggs to make an embryo to have a baby. The patient is the "recipient", and a woman whose eggs will be harvested is the "donor." The need for this aggressive treatment is determined by the reproductive endocrinologist (RE). The RE, also known as the fertility doctor, collaborates with other specialties in this type of treatment plan because it involves more layers than traditional IVF. A maternal-fetal medicine physician determines if the recipient (mostly the older woman) is healthy enough to carry a pregnancy. An attorney ensures the recipient reviews and signs a contract. (The donor also signs a contract, as described below.) The mental health specialist, such as a psychologist, evaluates the recipient to make sure she is psychologically stable to pursue having a baby who will not be genetically related.

Once these parts are glued together, the fertility specialist may move forward with the donor-matching process with a live donor or donor frozen eggs from an egg bank. Fresh donor eggs are retrieved from a younger woman who volunteers to donate her eggs to help another woman achieve motherhood. The donor is selected by profile from the infertility clinic's donor pool or a donor agency. This process is less tedious when using donor sperm. It takes invasive clinical procedures to prep and harvest eggs.

A donor egg treatment cycle is the most expensive infertility treatment. It can surpass more than twenty-five thousand dollars. Still, that price tag only covers the compensation for the donor's time, medical fees, and reproductive technology and medical facility use. A price tag is NOT associated with eggs' actual cost because that is "a donation". That donation births a family and future generations for the recipient.

When I meet with egg donors for an initial review of a treatment plan, I repeat my mantra, "We can never compensate you for your generosity and gift of your eggs to help another woman achieve motherhood. The fee offered to you by the recipient can only compensate for your time."

A typical fee to the donor is $8,000 per cycle; other clinics pay about the same, while donor agencies pay a bit lower but cover travel, meals, and accommodation if applicable. Most donors enter an egg donation program with altruistic motives: they are not interested in monetary gain alone but want to help others.

How Does the Egg Donor Treatment Work?

The egg donor needs daily injections to recruit the entire crop of eggs for her ovaries produces that month. The egg donor has frequent blood and ultrasound procedures during the injection (stimulation) phase. When her eggs are mature (after about ten days of being on daily injections), she is scheduled for egg retrieval two days later. The egg retrieval is a surgical procedure to remove many microscopic eggs from her ovaries. The entire donor-IVF cycle and procedures are essentially the same when women undergo IVF using their own eggs to have their own baby. Anonymous donors are only qualified to donate if they have an excellent egg reserve as measured by their blood work results of AMH and AFC.

Once the eggs are retrieved, they are no longer the donor's. They now belong to the recipient as per the contract both parties signed. The eggs get fertilized with the recipient's partner's sperm (or donor sperm if indicated) to form embryos.

One day after the retrieval and fertilization with sperm, the team determines the number of viable embryos (not every egg will fertilize successfully). The embryos are transferred to the recipient's uterus to help her achieve pregnancy. The embryo transfer can be done fresh, about 6 days later, or frozen, a month or more later.

Because donors tend to recruit many eggs, they may develop Ovarian Hyperstimulation Syndrome (OHSS). Its symptoms are shortness of breath, nausea, vomiting, feeling bloated, pain or tenderness in the ovarian area, and discomfort with urination. These symptoms may be mild to severe. There is also a risk of ovarian torsion (when an ovary twists on its own), which may result in the loss of an ovary, although this is not common. Providing there are no complications, the donor is monitored for about an hour after the egg retrieval procedure. The donor goes home with clinical guidance and her monetary compensation.

A donor can attempt several egg donations cycles per her lifetime, and this does not deplete her reserve if she wants to have children later in her fertile years.

For example, Giselle (fictious name) called my clinic to ask if she could have some of the eggs she donated thirteen years prior. Giselle was in her forties and having difficulties conceiving. She had a couple of successful donor egg cycles in her twenties, but it never crossed her mind that she would need help now. Unfortunately, Giselle experienced age-related decline in egg reserve and egg quality. She was even willing to ask the recipient of her eggs to donate an embryo; she thought that at least she could have a child with her own DNA. The fertility center could not honor her request because of a binding contract and an anonymous donor-recipient relationship.

Three Common Egg Donation Treatment Scenarios

Anonymous egg donation

Many medical centers in New York and other states have an anonymous egg donor program. Although the recipients of the donated eggs receive details about their donors' medical, ethnic, psychosocial, and academic backgrounds, they cannot see current photos or meet the donor. They must rely solely on the data presented by the infertility center, which often includes a celebrity-look-alike photo. Additionally, both donor and recipient must sign a contract that prevents them from obtaining identifying information that may be used for future contact by either party or potential offspring.

Partially known egg donor treatment plan

There are egg donor agencies that allow the recipient to see the donors' photos that are current and/or at different stages of their lives, and even have a web conference between recipients and donors without sharing other identifying information. Before making this critical and life-changing selection, women who want to see the donor's physical features and assess their skills and intelligence levels prefer using a partially known egg donor plan.

Working with an egg donor agency comes with additional challenges, including scheduling tests and monitoring promptly. This is even more challenging when selecting an egg donor from out-of-state within the USA or overseas. There may be immigration challenges and more financial expenses related to travel and accommodations if the donor lives far away or overseas.

Known Egg-Donor Treatment Plan

In this scenario, women and couples chose a family member as their egg donor. This type of donation, though done out of pure generosity and love, can become complicated. The treatment plan includes a thorough psychological screening of both donor and recipient. Before starting this treatment, the recipient and donor sign an iron-clad contract. No one wants their known donor to claim later that the baby belongs to her or seek to take the baby away from the recipient legally.

In some parts of the U.S. and the world, this type of known egg donor plan is forbidden. There are also the moral, psychological, and ethical aspects to overcome before and after embarking on such a journey.

Identical twin Maria came to the infertility clinic where I worked. At age 34, she had a history of severe endometriosis that required removal of one ovary and blocked fallopian tubes. She also had a quite diminished ovarian reserve because of the endometriosis and oophorectomy (removal of ovary). Maria got no embryos from two IVF cycles using autologous (her own eggs). Her best chance was to conceive using donor eggs. She felt an urgency to conceive as soon as possible since she faced the possibility of her endometriosis leading to loss of her second ovary and onset of menopause.

Maria's twin sister, Alissa, already had two children without difficulties. Alissa lovingly volunteered to donate her eggs to her sister. The treatment plan went smoothly except for the effort to coordinate their hectic travel schedules. Maria gave birth to her daughter using her sister's eggs and retained the embryos for more children.

Maria is the baby's mother by birth and legal rights, while Alissa is the aunt and DNA mother. Alissa said that there is nothing that she will not do for her sister Maria. Both their husbands were supportive. This was one of the most beautiful stories I have seen in the world of egg donation.

Embryo Donation

Most women and couples do not think they will ever need to decide to have a baby with someone else's embryos. This is the last method on anyone's mind. In this case, the baby will be devoid of the DNA from the adoptive parents. However, when a couple gets to this phase or potential plan, they have usually tried all other possible therapies. They are often depleted—emotionally, mentally, and financially. When this happens, the most important goal–having a baby–remains strong, propelling them to go this route.

An embryo donation cycle works like a frozen embryo transfer (FET) cycle and is much less expensive. The donated embryos are not purchased – they are usually gifts from a couple who have achieved the desired number of children. They have remaining embryos they do not want to destroy due to personal, psychological, and religious factors and beliefs. The recipient gets the embryos(s) transferred to her uterus, hopefully, gets pregnant, and delivers her baby. In most cases, these donations are also anonymous; the donating parents do not know the adoptive parents.

In another usual situation, Emily and Kris Burns could not conceive before they turned to embryo adoption. The embryo had been frozen for twenty years before the doctor implanted it in Emily's uterus. As Emily says, "He was just sitting there in a freezer waiting for someone to call him their own. Now he's our perfect little child." (Sechtin, 2020)

It is exceedingly rare that a "donor embryo" transaction happens between people who know each other. Only once in my career, and very recently, did I encounter such a plan. It involved a neighbor of one of my patients who generously donated her two remaining embryos who were cryopreserved at the same clinic. Susie, my 44-year-old patient, failed to conceive from a few IVF cycles with her own eggs. Her money was depleted; she took out a home equity loan, the pandemic happened, and she lost her job. Her husband's insurance did not offer fertility benefits, and out of much frustration, he walked out. She found so much compassion with her neighbor and hopes that she will be successful and that her husband will eventually return.

There are fewer legal stumbling blocks in the case of embryo adoption than traditional adoption of a baby.

The average pregnancy success rate using an adopted embryo is approximately 40%, slightly higher than the standard IVF implantation pregnancy success rate. This may be because donated embryos come from an already successful batch, and some may have undergone preimplantation genetic testing and shown to be chromosomally normal.

I was privileged to be the nurse in charge of the egg and embryo donation program of one of the most successful infertility clinics in the country that offered these services. I helped the adopted parents navigate this journey and visited them as new parents of babies from adopted embryos. The one significant factor that stood out with these new parents is how over-the-moon in love they are with their babies. All prior stigma, psychological, spiritual, and ethical concerns become overshadowed by the pure joy and fulfillment their babies brought.

One interesting sperm donation and egg donation case that I was involved with as a nurse was Andy and Holly's case. Holly's diagnosis was premature ovarian failure at age thirty-three, and she needed to get an egg donor. Andy's semen analysis was normal. As I was presenting the treatment protocol, synchronizing their plan with the anonymous egg donor, and conducting the injection class, I learned they were planning to use a sperm donor as well.

Of course, I asked what the reasoning behind it was, given that Andy had no sperm issues.

Andy responded with a first-of-a-kind rationale. Andy wanted to keep his DNA out of their child's conception out of empathy to his wife, who needed donor eggs. What was even more remarkable was that Holly's brother, David, would be the sperm donor. When I asked about the rationale behind that, they told me that they wanted the baby/babies still to have Holly's DNA as part of their family. Of course, the legal contacts and psychological clearance had to get done before they could move forward.

When all the preliminaries were completed, Holly announced that she wanted to be far away when the donor would start the treatment cycle. She only wanted one phone call when the embryos were ready, even after the pre-implantation genetic screening results were available.

More than a year later, someone touched me on my shoulder in the shopping mall and could not stop raving about her baby. Holly's iPhone had the most beautiful mommy and baby boy pictures. She said that except for a few weeks of postpartum depression, her life has completely changed for the best.

Gestational Carrier and Surrogacy

Gestational surrogacy is a solution when a couple is missing the essential ingredient of a uterus or life-threatening complications if she carries the pregnancy. The embryos created by sperm and egg are implanted into the woman who will carry the baby to term (delivery). This is the most common form of surrogacy and often needed when there is an underlying medical problem that puts the biological mother at risk if she carries a pregnancy or does not have a uterus. Each year there were approximately 750 cases of gestational surrogacy in the USA before 2015. Among them are a few celebrities: Kim Kardashian and Sarah Jessica Parker.

The surrogacy rate is growing, and one of the reasons for the increase is the rights, openness, and access to procreation of the LGBTQ populations. CNN correspondent Anderson Cooper's story is an example. A gay male, Anderson used a surrogate to achieve fatherhood. According to Heather Jacobson, "Gestational surrogacy via egg donation in U.S.-based infertility clinics is understood to be an increasingly popular route to planned fatherhood for gay men able to afford these services" (A limited market: the recruitment of gay men as surrogacy clients by the infertility industry in the USA, 2018).

There was also an increase in foreigners coming to the USA for this type of treatment – although this has been on the decline with more restrictive immigration criteria (Perkins, K. et al, 2016). Surrogacy is a popular option for gay men who want to be biologically connected to their children and for lesbian couples (although less needed) who are unable to conceive or carry a pregnancy on their own (Gay Surrogacy – Surrogacy for the LGBT Couples).

Gestational surrogacy also allows male partners to have children. In an unusual story, Cecile, a 61-year-old mother in Nebraska, carried a baby to term for her son Matthew and his husband, Elliott. Matthew's sister donated the egg; Elliott provided the sperm. After Cecile agreed to be the gestational carrier, she underwent hormone treatment to restart her menstrual periods. All it took was one embryo transfer before she began carrying her granddaughter, who was born healthy (Steussey, 2019).

IVF is part of the process to create the embryos. The surrogate or gestational carrier will undergo the embryo transfer – typically a frozen embryo transfer (FET) procedure. Depending on the state, surrogacy may not be permitted, and when it is, FDA regulations govern this process.

Marsha had an emergency hysterectomy when she delivered her son six years ago. She and Bill, her husband, were planning to have at least three kids because they each came from a family of three. As her pregnancy progressed, she learned she had placenta accrete, a serious pregnancy condition that occurs when the placenta grows too deeply into the uterine wall and becomes challenging to detach at childbirth. This condition can lead to life-threatening bleeding and in most cases a hysterectomy is eminent and lifesaving.

In Marsha's case, she needed an emergency hysterectomy to stop the bleeding. Marsha and Bill were terrified; in that sheer moment of panic, they didn't realize that their dream for more kids was gone with the uterus. All they wanted was for this nightmare to be over so they could be parents to their newborn.

Placenta accrete is the second most common indication for an emergency hysterectomy at childbirth. It occurs in 75% (seven out of every ten) of women who had a prior cesarean delivery (c-section) or dilatation and curettage (D&C). Unfortunately for Marsha, she had a history of two D&Cs. Although she was at risk of developing placenta accrete, she didn't fully comprehend the full risk until her son's delivery. When Joshua was 3-years-old, Bill and Marsha wished for more kids – but how can they do that without a uterus?

At the time of this writing, Bill and Marsha had completed grieving the loss of Marsha's reproductive ability and were getting care in a New York IVF clinic so they could create their embryos.

Both Bill and Marsha work for an employer whose healthcare insurance policy provides surrogacy coverage of up to twenty thousand dollars. The caveat is that the plan only pays for the healthcare bills for the surrogate/gestation carrier but will not cover the surrogate's monetary compensation.

In April 2020, the NYS governor signed a law allowing Compensated Surrogacy and Gestational (services) in New York. The law established a minimum compensation between $30,000-$40,000, plus additional compensation and benefits for milestones along their journey (Surrogacy Laws in New York, n.d). Surrogacy can cost over 100,000 dollars, including surrogate compensation. Some insurance carriers may cover some of these expenses.

This is a milestone for people in New York. Infertility doctors are bracing for the flood of requests involving surrogacy in 2021 when this law takes full effect, and the pandemic is hopefully behind us.

Although this law was enacted April 2020, the COVID-19 Pandemic put a screeching halt to moving forward. Surrogacy contracts may begin on February 15, 2021, allowing New Yorkers to compensate a surrogate legally. The state's paid surrogacy law includes the Surrogates' Bill of Rights, the strongest protections for surrogates in the nation. The surrogate must be at least 21-years-old.

Only altruistic surrogacy was permitted before this new law. New York has finally implemented this much-needed law, and it is a victory for women who must have a surrogate because of a medical diagnosis.

Until the law passed, a woman who required a surrogate in New York had to ask a family member to volunteer. For example, the Washington Post published a beautiful story of a mother who was her daughter's gestational carrier. Julie Loving, 51 years old from Long Island, carried her daughter, Brianna Lockwood, and husband's Aaron Lockwood's baby to birth. Brianna battled infertility for years (Page, 2020). Her only option was IVF to create embryos and then have someone else carry her baby. In the end, her mother did the honors. Of course, in addition to signing the legal agreements, at age 51, she had to be evaluated by a Maternal Fetal Medicine physician to be deemed healthy to carry a pregnancy to term without jeopardizing her own health. This is the beautiful gift of altruistic gestational carrier/surrogacy.

These states are considered surrogacy-friendly, according to Surrogate.com:

- California
- Connecticut
- Delaware
- District of Columbia
- Maine
- New Hampshire
- New York
- Nevada
- Oregon
- Rhode Island
- Washington

Chapter 3

Pre-Implantation Genetic Testing

"Will my baby be normal?" Every parent thinks about this. The answers lay in comprehensive chromosome screening (CCS) and pre-implantation genetic testing (PGT). Pre-implantation genetic testing of embryos before transferring them into the uterus is more commonplace today. These tests are only done when a patient goes through IVF.

This chapter sheds light on the types of pre-implantation genetic testing of embryos (performed with IVF), their indications, benefits, and implications. It also gives an idea of other fetal screening and testing ordered during pregnancy – especially for those conceptions that happened naturally or by artificial insemination (AI aka IUI).

Genetic Mutations: Testing the Parents

There are two types of genetic mutations: dominant and recessive. During the diagnostic phase of infertility workup a simple blood test on the parents identifies if one or both are carriers of a *recessive* genetic mutation or a *dominant* genetic mutation. If they are each carriers of the same recessive mutation or either or both have a dominant trait, it puts their offspring at risk for a genetic disorder.

If only one of them is a recessive disorder carrier, there is typically no concern that a child would be afflicted with a genetic disease. At most, a child may have just the carrier status. If there is a risk of passing on a genetic disease to an offspring, pre-implantation embryo testing is paramount.

There are three kinds of basic pre-implantation testing of the embryo under the term PGT (pre-implantation genetic testing): PGT-A, PGT-M, and PGT-SR.

In all three, the embryologist biopsies the embryo to get a tiny bit of tissue for testing. Depending on the type of test needed the result may be available within 1-6 weeks. While the biopsies are prepared and examined during this timeframe, the embryos are cryopreserved (frozen) in liquid nitrogen and can be kept for many years until transferred to the uterus for potential pregnancy.

How Cells Divide and Separate after Fertilization

Although both sperm and eggs have potential to cause a malfunction, the aged egg has a much greater potential of doing so; hence most genetic errors are because of older eggs (Alexander Webster and Melina Schuh, 2016). A human has 23 pairs of chromosomes (46 total). One chromosome of each pair comes from each of two parents (male and female). Twenty-two pairs are called "autosomes" and look the same, while the twenty-third pair is the "sex" chromosomes and looks different.

The cells of the new embryo go through a mitosis (dividing and multiplying) to form identical duplicates, but if there is a "mis-allocation" of chromosomes during this process, aneuploidy result (an abnormal number of chromosomes).

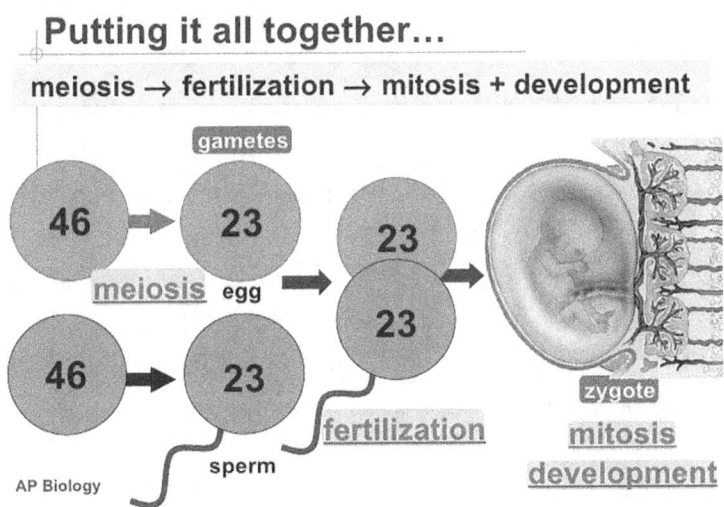

Source: google.com/search?q=meiosis+fertilization+mitosis&tbm=isch&ved=2ahUKEwiUI57EnuLsAhVFPN8KHYMrB2UQ2-cCegQIABAA&oq=-meiosis+

Pre-implantation Genetic Screening (PGS) of the Embryo: PGT-A

Recessive gene mutation

PGT-A is pre-implantation genetic testing on embryos using a scientific technology of ruling out chromosomal abnormalities (aneuploidy). If an embryo is normal, it is an "euploid". If it is abnormal, it is an "aneuploid" or "aneuploidy."

PGT-A testing is often incorporated into the IVF treatment cycles to decrease the probability of transferring an abnormal embryo into the uterus. When an embryo is chromosomally abnormal, it often leads to failed implantation or early miscarriage. PGT-A helps the clinicians select normal embryos which are most likely to result in a successful outcome.

A parent-to-be may request genetic screening for family balancing because the result also defines whether the embryo is a male (**XY** chromosomes) or a female (**XX** chromosomes). Although not all the time, parents want to know the sex of the embryo, so tha they have the opportunity of deciding whether to transfer a male or female embryo. (There are ethical issues associated with making decisions based on the embryo's sex, as I cover later.)

An inherent recessive genetic disease of a child occurs when both parents are *carriers* of a *recessive* genetic mutation such as cystic fibrosis (CF), spinal muscular atrophy (SMA), Gaucher, etc. Together, they have a **25%** risk of having a baby with the disease, 25% of having an unaffected baby, and **50%** of having a baby who is a carrier (see image below).

A *recessive* genetic mutation such as cystic fibrosis requires binding to another CF gene to manifest the disease. A "carrier" does not have the disease and is not symptomatic. However, if both parents are CF carriers, they can pass this gene on to an offspring. An offspring can then inherit the two CF copies ogf the gene and become afflicted with

CF disease. Similarly, an offspring can inherit the CF from one parent and just be a carrier but not afflicted with the disease. During mitosis, chromosomes XX and XY give four variations. (See diagram.)

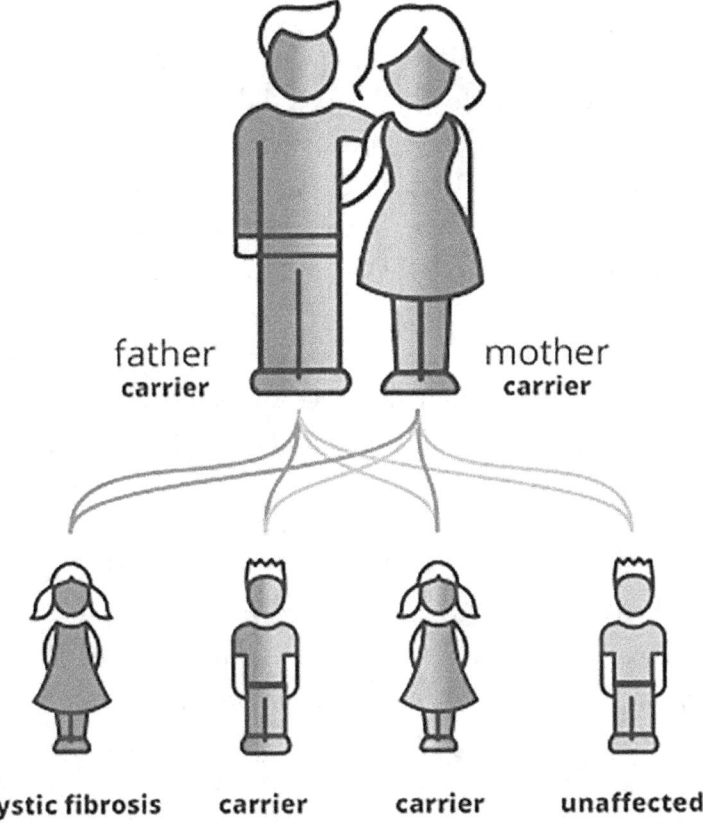

A genetic panel is a simple blood test done during the infertility workup on each parent to identify their genetic status. If only one potential parent is a carrier while the other is not, there is no risk of the offspring being afflicted. In addition to cystic fibrosis, over two hundred genetic mutations have been identified so far, and more continue to be discovered. If there is a risk of passing on a genetic disease (recessive or dominant) preconception genetic counseling by genetic specialist is vital before moving forward with IVF.

Testing revealed Irina was spinal muscular atrophy (SMA) carrier, but her husband, George, did not undergo testing. They reasoned, "The test costs a lot of money," and their insurance did not cover it. They reckoned "what are the chances we would be both carriers?" They became pregnant with twins through IVF and were elated.

However, at 18 weeks of pregnancy, their happiness turned to horror. An ultrasound revealed the babies were afflicted with spinal muscular atrophy – the number one genetic cause of death in infants.

Irina and George were devastated. Their clinicians recommended termination of the pregnancy. As their nurse, my heart broke for them. I watched and listened as they replayed their miscalculation of the probability of this genetic tragedy. Later, blood tests confirmed that George, too, was a carrier of SMA.

Irina and George spent over sixty thousand dollars (U.S.) and several years on IVF with Irina's eggs. Emotionally and psychologically exhausted, they took a break to heal. When Irina was age 42, they returned to the clinic and learned that Irina's egg reserve had declined drastically, and the only chance at parenthood would be through donor eggs or donor embryos. They relived the pain of taking chances all over again. As I worked with this couple, I watched how they left all the decision-making to the clinicians (the doctor, the nurse, and the embryologist). They did not trust their own decision-making ability anymore. It was sad to watch and listen. At the end of it all, Irina used IVF and a donor egg. She delivered a gorgeous baby boy. He brought peace, joy, and inner healing to them.

Reproductive specialists often suggest genetic screening for women older than 35 years, women who have had failed implantation, and for other medical or genetic reasons. These are a few common reasons PGT-A (PGS) is performed:

1. Advanced reproductive age: As women age, the quality and quantity of their eggs declines.
2. Recurrent pregnancy loss: The test is completed for those who suffer recurrent pregnancy losses (RPL), which is usually a result of chromosomal abnormalities that lead to miscarriages up to about 20 weeks of gestation. Although losses may result from an ectopic (tubal) pregnancy or a biochemical pregnancy, they do not get labeled under the diagnosis of RPL because the pregnancy is not a "clinical" one.
3. Another reason for PGS testing is trisomy, a condition in which an extra copy of a chromosome is present in the cell nuclei causing developmental abnormalities. A trisomy is the **most** frequently detected anomaly – in over 60% of pregnancy anomalies. This abnormality can be detected by conducting

genetic testing on products of conception (POC) from a clinical pregnancy loss. The pregnancy tissue typically is obtained from a dilation and curettage (D&C) procedure of that miscarriage.

Pre-implantation Genetic Screening (PGS) of the Embryo: PGT-SR

PGS and PGT-SR are essentially the same. This is the "screening" of the embryos created from IVF to determine if any of them have abnormally arranged or sized chromosomes. When there are chromosome structural rearrangements, one or more embryos(s) may have extra or missing genetic material. This typically results in early pregnancy loss. (PGT, what does it all mean? 2018)

Pre-implantation Genetic Diagnosis (PGD) of the Embryo: PGT-M

Dominant gene mutation

The PGT-M test looks for monogenic disorders involving a single gene known to be "dominant' or "X-linked". These genes are associated with inherited disorders, such as Fragile-X, Huntington's disease, and a few more. In contrast to PGT-A, the PGT-M test on the embryos is specific to a "dominant" genetic disorder. The intent is to avoid transferring an embryo afflicted with a specific genetic disorder. When a parent has a disease associated with a dominant gene there is a genetic concern or family history that predisposes **50%** of a couple's offspring to the genetic disease. The PGD also referred to PGT-M (M for monogenic/single gene defect) testing procedure is more in-depth, takes longer to test, and identifies dominant gene defects within embryos before implantation. It takes only one parent with a dominant mutation to pass the disease to a child. The father is a carrier for one dominant "mutated" gene in the diagram below, while the mother does not carry a dominant "mutated" gene. Unlike the 25% risk associated with the "recessive" trait, the risk associated with dominant is **50%**.

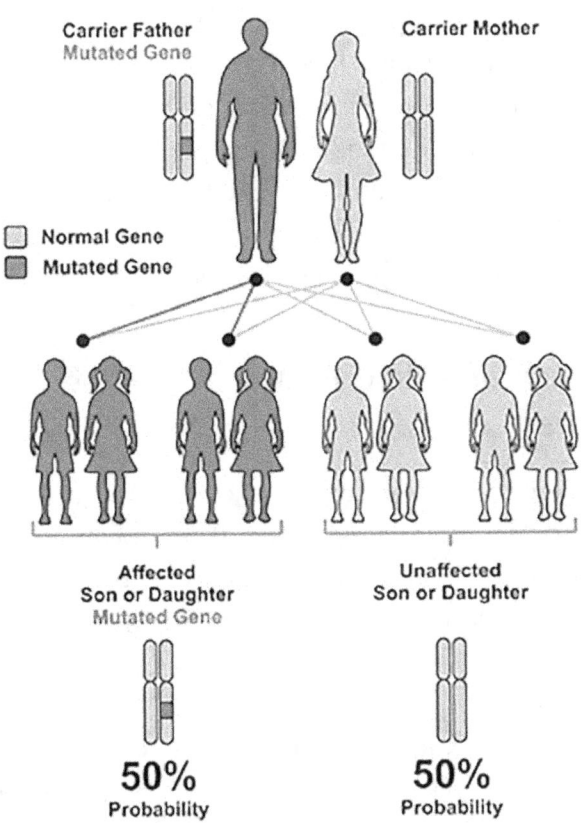

Source: https://www.niddk.nih.gov/health-information/diabetes/overview/what-is-diabetes/monogenic-neonatal-mellitus-mody

A dominant gene mutation creates a risk for a genetically abnormal fetus when only one parent has a mutation that, by itself, can cause disease in the fetus where abnormal genes dominate. It is possible that a genetic disease can also occur as a new condition in a child when neither parent has the abnormal gene. A typical example is Huntington's disease.

The fertility doctors and many reproductive facilities across the country partner with several reference laboratories that perform pre-implantation genetic testing on embryos. Leading laboratories are Igenomix, Cooper Genomics, and Natera. Some insurance carriers cover the biopsy procedure and/or testing of the embryos. Insurance may also select one or more testing laboratory as in-network. It is important that patients and providers understand the insurance benefits and when they need to pay privately.

Situations in Which PGT or CCG Are Not Indicated

It is unnecessary to undergo genetic testing when a biochemical pregnancy loss occurs after a positive urinary pregnancy test (human chorionic gonadotropin - hCG) or a positive blood serum -hCG before ultrasound or histological verification. Biochemical pregnancies are often missed, especially in women who are not planning to become pregnant and may think that the late bleeding is a delayed menstrual period. In the case of a biochemical pregnancy, there is no opportunity to collect the products of conception for testing, and as a result, no chance to examine any tissue.

Ectopic pregnancy losses are a result of fallopian tube issues. Scarring or blockages in the fallopian tube may result in the pregnancy getting stuck in the tubes. Fertilization takes place in the fallopian tubes where the egg and sperm meet. As the embryonic cells multiply and divide, the clump/ball of cells travels down to the uterus and finds a spot on the uterine wall (womb) to implant and grow – becoming a baby. Scarring or blockage in the fallopian tubes often results from pelvic inflammatory disease (PID) caused by two sexually transmitted diseases: gonorrheal and chlamydia, endometriosis, cysts, or hydrosalpinx. The tube ruptures because it is not wide enough to accommodate the developing zygote to embryo.

Benefits of Comprehensive Chromosome Screening (CCS) and PGT

When the indication for pre-implantation genetic screening is to rule out abnormal embryos, it is usually medically necessary and understandable. But many, including clinicians agree there are ethical and moral concerns when a couple chooses testing for the sole purpose of sex selection and family balancing, referred to as biological engineering.

Sarah (fictitious name) had four sons and only wanted a daughter to result from her next pregnancy. She attempted two IVF with PGS but created only male embryos. To my shock and the clinicians' concerns, she requested that all seven of her male normal embryos be discarded. Additionally, she was quite upset and demanded to be fully reimbursed for IVF and PGS because she did not have a female embryo. The facility's reputation was at stake, and it was not willing to continue IVF with PGS with these demands. Neither could it reimburse her for exceptional services that were already rendered. She relented and made a third IVF/PGS attempt.

On her third attempt, Sarah did not want to know if she had a female embryo or not. She dictated that the doctor proceeds with an embryo transfer procedure regardless but only transfer an embryo if it was female. She was willing to pay privately for the FET cycle to the end and have a negative pregnancy test than be told that she has failed to create a female embryo. Due to ethical concerns, the clinic could not agree with this demand, and Sarah did not continue there as a patient.

For women who conceive naturally or with IUI procedure, several other tests can detect abnormalities. These include the MS-AFP (maternal serum alpha-fetoprotein), nuchal translucency (NT), amniocentesis, CVS (chorionic villus sampling), and a Level II Ultrasound. These tests are done in early pregnancy (between 10-20 weeks of pregnancy) to detect anomalies such as Down's syndrome, spina bifida, cystic fibrosis, and other disorders.

- **MS-AFP** - The alpha-fetoprotein test measures high and low levels of alpha-fetoprotein. The results are combined with the mother's age and ethnicity to assess potential genetic disorders' probabilities. High levels of AFP may suggest the developing baby has a neural tube defect such as spina bifida or anencephaly. Because the result is based on the combined data plotted on a graph, follow-up tests such as amniocentesis is needed to confirm the result.

- **Nuchal Translucency** – This test uses ultrasound to measure the fluid buildup's thickness at the back of the developing baby's neck. If this area is thicker than normal, it can be an early sign of Down syndrome, trisomy 18, or heart problems. Here again, a confirmatory test is needed.

- **Amniocentesis** – A sample of the amniotic fluid helps to diagnose specific health problems in an unborn baby. These include genetic disorders, which are often caused by changes (mutations) in certain genes. The test detects cystic fibrosis and Tay-Sachs disease. This test can confirm most disorders but cannot detect structural birth defects — such as heart malformations or a cleft lip or palate. Under sterile conditions the doctor uses a long needle to penetrate through the pregnant abdomen to withdraw fluid from the amniotic sac for testing.

- **Chorionic villus sampling** - This transcervical procedure is performed by inserting a thin plastic tube through the vagina and cervix to reach the placenta. The healthcare provider uses ultrasound images to help guide the tube into the best area for sampling. A small sample of chorionic villus (placental) tissue is then removed for testing. The test detects chromosomal conditions, such as Down's syndrome and other genetic conditions, such as cystic fibrosis. It can also tell the gender of the fetus. As with amniocentesis, there is a risk of infection to the fetus because foreign microbes can be introduced into the sterile environment of the amniotic space of the fetus. This risk can be fatal.

- **Level II Ultrasound** – The ultrasound is done between 18-20 weeks of pregnancy and is like a standard ultrasound. The difference is that the doctor will get more detailed information on anatomical structure. The doctor may focus on specific parts of the baby's body, such as his or her brain, heart, or other organs. Women may get a targeted ultrasound in their second trimester. This ultrasound can detect structural anomalies such as cleft palate, and genetic disorder such as spinal muscular atrophy.

CHAPTER 4

COST AND INSURANCE COVERAGE

"How much will it cost us?" Not too long ago, the cost of infertility treatment was totally out-of-pocket cost to patients. Those days are behind us now because most infertility-related therapies are covered by health insurance. There is no federal law requiring insurance carriers to provide coverage for infertility care, but state mandates require some coverage. So far, seventeen states within the USA have enacted laws that offer some level of coverage using specific guidelines.

Although these laws may be different, each either has the mandate to *cover* or a mandate to *offer* care, as you will see in the table below. Generally, public insurance does not provide infertility benefits, but private insurances do. Private insurances fall under one of these three categories: commercial insurance, self-insurance groups where employers pay benefit claims directly rather than using an outside insurance carrier such as Blue Cross Blue Shield (BCBS), and non-profit insurance companies. In instances where employers pay claims directly, they may still hire an outside carrier like BCBS, Cigna, and so on to serve as the benefits manager. These benefit managers dictate the policy and determine covered services.

The health insurance policy is an agreement between the patient's employer and the insurance company. This agreement lists all the stipulations. Additionally, to access this coverage, you or your employer would pay or share the cost of a fixed premium each year to an insurer. There may also be a copay per visit or a deductible the patient is responsible for upfront before the health plan pays its portion.

Another stipulation to consider is whether, in addition to in-network services, the plan also allows out-of-network (OON) coverage and in-for-out (IFO) coverage. IFO applies when a plan may approve services at an OON provider or facility if in-network providers and facilities are *not* within a limited number of miles from the patient's home.

Prospective parents must understand the details of their health plans as it relates to infertility. Coverage varies significantly and may significantly differ from one employer to another, even with the same insurance company as BCBS, Cigna, Aetna, etc.

Thoroughly review and seek clarification about a plan's provisions, paying attention to specific covered services. Examine the criteria that you must meet, services that are excluded, and restrictions related to infertility diagnosis, treatment plan, and other related services.

Although the health plan administrator will provide prospective parents with a copy of the plan's Summary Plan

Description (SPD), the language is often difficult to decipher. An employee may need to call the health plan to understand the covered services.

As discussed in Chapter 1, an example is a diagnosis of infertility, which is necessary for many insured patients to take advantage of the infertility benefits.

In collaboration with the health plan, some employers may include an organization that specializes in infertility to assist their members in understanding and navigating through this tedious aspect of their journey. Specialized infertility nurses staff such an organization like Women Integrated Network (WIN-Healthcare) and Progeny. An infertility nurse would be able to help members to:

- assist the patient in interpreting the details of the infertility coverage,
- provider clarity where there may be confusion,
- provide nursing support and guidance,
- process authorization for treatment and medications,
- collaborate with the member's provider and specialty pharmacies, and
- even assist when there are conflicts related to claims, reimbursement, and overall coverage.

Nurses help patients receive adequate education so that they can take full advantage of covered benefits. Women's Integrated Network (WIN) is an organization that tops the chart among a very few of its type. It has the best of the specialized infertility nurses in the country. The members who work for companies that collaborated with WIN are happier because their employees (members) get the expert guidance and support they need out of the covered benefits.

- According to recent data, a basic IVF cycle can cost over twelve thousand dollars. When other components such as intracytoplasmic sperm injection (ICSI) or assisted hatching are warranted, the cost can increase by a few thousand dollars. (Hatching occurs when the embryo breaks out of the protective shell that surrounds the ball of fertilized cells. The embryologist may need to make a small opening in the embryo's outer shell before it is placed into the woman's body by the physician. The hope is that assisted hatching might help the embryo to break out of its shell, expand, implant, and lead to pregnancy.)

- Additionally, if portions of the facility, such as the embryology lab and surgical suites are out-of-network with a health plan that only covers in-network services, the cost becomes more insurmountable. However, although a still daunting investment, clients count their blessings knowing that they would have had to pay a hundred percent of the treatment cost in the recent past. Now that has changed - thanks to many employers who have become more vested in their employees' happiness. Coverage varies from one employer to another regarding what infertility services they choose to include in their health packages. One employer may pay for basic coverage, while another may pay for more.

- Thanks to research, science, and technology, we know the etiology of infertility is equally a male issue as it is a female. Given the high percentage of women in the workforce today, employers with a sense and fairness include infertility care in their employee benefits package. When employees are satisfied with a company, their productivity levels increase, hence the company's success.

Most insurance will not cover some PGT testing unless clinically indicated, such as in the case of a trisomy. Few insurance plans will cover the embryos' biopsy procedure for PGT-A in women older than 35 years. Older women have a greater likelihood of chromosomally abnormal embryos related to egg quality.

The insurance carrier may exclude paying for treatment for women who have had more than two clinical miscarriages. (A clinical miscarriage occurs when a pregnancy ultrasound reveals a fetus in the uterus or histological evidence through tissue testing confirms the presence of pregnancy tissue.)

When testing shows a chromosomal abnormality, the insurance may cover PGT-A in the IVF treatment cycles. Still, when there is no histological evidence of abnormality, most insurances will not cover the cost. The patient pays privately/out-of-pocket, which varies from $350 for biopsy of each embryo or $2500 per batch of over eight embryos depending on the provider's pay schedule. The lab testing fees also cost an equivalent amount.

Some states within the USA mandated health insurance must cover infertility treatment. Below is a table with some examples of variation by state.

State	State's Definition of Infertility	Examples of the State's Mandates
Arkansas	The patient and her spouse must have at least a 2-year history of unexplained infertility OR infertility must be associated with at least one of the following: endometriosis, DES exposure, blocked or surgically removed fallopian tubes that are not the result of voluntary sterilization, abnormal male factors contributing to infertility to receive coverage. The patient's eggs must be fertilized with her spouse's sperm. Using donor sperm will bar IVF coverage. The patient must prove her inability to obtain successful pregnancy through any lesser costly infertility treatments covered by insurance.	All individual and group (employer) insurance policies that provide maternity benefits must cover in-vitro fertilization (IVF). HMOs are exempt from this law in Arkansas. The lifetime maximum of coverage for infertility treatment is $15,000. IVF procedures must be performed at a facility licensed or certified by the state and conform to the American College of Obstetricians and Gynecologists' (ACOG) and the American Society of Reproductive Medicine's (ASRM) guidelines.

Cost and Insurance Coverage

State	State's Definition of Infertility	Examples of the State's Mandates
California	Infertility means the presence of a demonstrated condition recognized by a physician and surgeon as a cause of infertility or the inability to conceive a pregnancy or carry a pregnancy to a live birth after a year or more of regular sexual relations without contraception.	Requires group insurers to offer coverage of infertility treatment, except IVF. Employers may choose whether or not to include infertility coverage as part of their employee health benefits package.
Illinois	Infertility means the inability to conceive after one year of unprotected sexual intercourse or the inability to sustain a successful pregnancy. Infertility means the inability to conceive after one year of unprotected sexual intercourse or the inability to sustain a successful pregnancy.	Group insurers and HMOs that provide pregnancy-related coverage must provide infertility treatment including, but not limited to a diagnosis of infertility, IVF, uterine embryo lavage, embryo transfer, artificial insemination, GIFT, ZIFT, low tubal ovum transfer. Employers with fewer than 25 employees do not have to provide coverage. It does not require religious employers to cover infertility treatment.

State	State's Definition of Infertility	Examples of the State's Mandates
Maryland	The patient and the patient's spouse must have a history of infertility for 2 years. The infertility is associated with one of the following: endometriosis, DES exposure, blocked or surgically removed fallopian tubes, abnormal male factors contributing to infertility.	Individual and group insurance policies that provide pregnancy-related benefits must cover the cost of 3 IVFs per live birth. Lifetime maximum of $100,000. IVF procedures must be performed at clinics that conform to ASRM and ACOG Guidelines.
New York	Infertility means a disease or condition characterized by the incapacity to impregnate another person or to conceive, defined by the failure to establish a clinical pregnancy after twelve months of regular, unprotected sexual intercourse or therapeutic donor insemination, or after six months of regular, unprotected sexual intercourse or therapeutic donor insemination for a female thirty-five years of age or older. Earlier evaluation and treatment may be warranted based on an individual's medical history or physical findings.	Group policies must provide diagnostic tests and procedures that include such a hysterosalpingogram (HSG), semen analysis, blood test, ultrasound.

State	State's Definition of Infertility	Examples of the State's Mandates
Texas	If an employer chooses to offer the benefit, patients must meet the following: the patient or spouse is the policyholder; the patient's eggs must be fertilized with her spouse's sperm; the patient and the patient's spouse have a history of infertility of at least five continuous years or associated with endometriosis, DES, blockage of or surgical removal of one or both fallopian tubes or oligospermia, the patient has been unable to attain a pregnancy through less costly treatment covered under their policy.	Requires group insurers to offer coverage of IVF. Employers may choose whether or not to include infertility coverage as part of their employee health benefits package.

As you can see from the examples above, many states provide coverage but do so on a limited basis. For example, New York State recently mandated health insurances to cover basic infertility treatment. Options include monitored timed intercourse (TIC) cycle and artificial insemination (intrauterine inseminations.) New York City employees are now able to get unlimited IUI cycles covered when they meet the criteria. However, that does not apply to more invasive infertility treatments such as IVF, donor egg IVF, and surrogacy. For a woman or couple to have IVF coverage, donor egg IVF, and surrogacy, the employer will need to purchase advanced type coverage for its employees.

An example: if an infertile woman or couple works for the City of New York – e.g, teachers, police officers, firefighters, New York City as an employer will currently pay for three ART cycles (a combination of IVF with or without fresh embryo transfer, or stand-alone FET cycle) minus deductible and copay. Even with this generous coverage – something unheard of in recent years – there are restrictions to its plan through Anthem. In contrast, other institutions' employees may pay up to a dollar limit ranging from five thousand to one hundred thousand dollars per lifetime.

To contrast, employees of a major bank (name withheld) puts no limit on the number of IVF cycles an employee needs to have as long as their criteria are met, and the treatment plan makes clinical sense. At the same time, another similar institution may cover up to fifty thousand dollars max with similar clinical criteria.

An IVF cycle involves ovarian stimulation, fertilization by insemination (in the absence of a male factor), or intracytoplasmic sperm injection (**ICSI** – in the presence of a male factor), assisted hatching when applicable, and an embryo transfer. But if an employee of NYC plans to do PGT testing on her embryos or cannot – for some reason or the other – do a fresh embryo transfer (5-6 days after fertilization), she potentially forfeits the coverage of that embryo transfer. She must receive the transfer within a limited time frame of the egg retrieval.

In PGT testing, ovarian hyperstimulation syndrome (OHSS), a fresh transfer, cannot be performed. Hence, the patient loses that opportunity for the embryo transfer within that covered IVF cycle. Per a few employers' criteria, she may not regain that coverage of an embryo transfer when it's time for it and may have to utilize one of her FET coverage. In other words, where she would have had a total of three embryo transfer procedures, she now has two.

Additionally, there may be an age restriction with some infertility coverage where an infertile woman cannot utilize the available infertility coverage if she is over a certain age. Most other plans do not have this age criterion. These restrictions and/or criteria can change when the plan renews. The employers hold the key to any changes as they adjust the criterion as they please.

Because we compare infertility coverage and what employers allow their employees to have, some may not be able to access the infertility benefit if they are not proven to have an infertility diagnosis.

One category of patients affected by these criteria is those who have not tried to become pregnant with a male partner. Those are single females or same-sex female couples needing to use donor sperm. If a heterosexual couple has not attempted to become pregnant in the traditional way, they cannot readily use their infertility benefit. On the other hand, if a single female or same-sex female has not tried and failed to become pregnant with donor sperm insemination, they cannot readily use their infertility benefit. Some insurance plans may, however, waive this criterion.

A single patient with normal egg reserve, open fallopian tubes, and no other infertility diagnosis would need to pay out of pocket for a specified number of donor sperm insemination cycles before accessing her infertility benefit. If she does not get pregnant, she may then be allowed to access her coverage.

Although some employers may have a cap on the number of IVF cycles an employee can have, they may take the limit off the number of frozen embryo transfer (FET) cycles she can receive. For example, if an employee of those companies needs IVF and ends up with excess embryos, she can do as many FETs as possible she likes up until the last of her three covered IVF cycles. The caveat to this criterion is that she utilizes ALL her normal frozen embryos before she can access a subsequent IVF cycle.

While some plans require that genetic screening on embryos follow medical policy (see Chapter 3), some employers waive this policy. Additionally, other employers may have different benefits designs and allow pre-implantation genetic screening if a woman is older than 35 years old or has suffered two or more miscarriages. The employer's goal is to increase the productivity and quality of work-life of their employees put out. If the employees are happy, they will show gratitude and loyalty to the employer.

Employers of corporations may include a set amount of dollars for fertility treatments in their employees' health benefits package. The employer gets to dictate which infertility services they will subsidize. Some employees may have a cap on the dollar amount, while others may have a cap on the number and type of treatment cycles they would cover. These benefits are bought by the employers but administered by the health plan. As you can see in the table above, state mandates must be adhered to and what an employer may allot towards infertility services for employers.

Chapter 5

Navigating the Multi-layer and Complicated Journey of Infertility

To successfully navigate the infertility world, a woman and her partner (if applicable) need all the tips available and set in motion the wheels for this journey. They also need to engage all needed tools and available resources, including clinical and non-clinical, to intelligently allocate energy towards and stay on this journey for the shortest time possible until success.

The couple benefits from understanding their fertility, diagnoses, treatment plans, and the financial costs. They must also be willing to unravel and expose issues shrouded in secrecy and be ready to deal with potential setbacks.

There are many layers to get through in the world of infertility, and sometimes peeling these layers away can become painful. Initially, it's the shock that you cannot have children naturally or of your own. It's the sting and stigma that seem to be the ever-present company on this journey – from trying to understand the diagnosis to finding a doctor to comprehend the medical terminology. The couple also confronts the financial affordability, let alone the psychological, emotional, spiritual, and ethical factors that pop up along the way.

Many couples locate an infertility doctor by asking for recommendations from another reputable doctor or colleague. The health plan's list of specialists may not always be the best for them. It is not a good idea to try to find a doctor on Yelp or the internet.

Get a second opinion if you doubt the first one, even if that means you may need to pay out of pocket. During those visits, you should also be able to get an overview of the clinic's atmosphere (warm or cold in terms of how you are treated) and each clinic's operating style. These are essential factors that impact your confidence and comfort level with that doctor and the clinic staff, and these factors can help manage your expectations. Ask questions about their success rates given your diagnoses. The American Society of Reproductive Medicine (ASRM) and Society of Reproductive Technology (SART) have valuable information about each infertility clinic and its annual success date.

Tips From an Infertility Nurse

The financial aspect is a significant factor and is often complicated. If you have infertility insurance coverage, get to know the details. You can best maximize the benefits within your health plan packages when you understand essential inclusions and exclusions, in-network versus out-of-network information. Understand what you need to do to access the fullest of benefits.

If your health insurance does not cover medications or only covers a small fraction of the toral, ask the specialty pharmacies about discount programs or out-of-pocket costs as there may be significantly reduced prices.

When required, set aside money through flex spending or health saving account through your payroll contributions – these are pre-tax dollars that can be used for out-of-pocket expenses. Talk to your provider's financial advisor about sources available to subsidize the cost of treatment.

Many patients may not have the luxury of infertility coverage within their health plans. When they do, the benefits can be used up before they fulfill their goals of family building. Some organizations may assist with loans and grants for fertility treatment if qualified.

WIN-Healthcare (formerly known as WIN-Fertility) has a DTC (direct-to-consumer) program which offers a "bundled package" that includes the treatment and prescriptions, and a prescription-only program that can be a more affordable option. WIN-Healthcare works with infertility clinics across the country.

Incorporate healthy lifestyle choices and relaxation techniques such as acupuncture, massage therapy, mindful meditations, and other alternative approaches, as mentioned in Chapter 24. Seek counseling if needed and talk to a close friend or relative you trust. Of course, speak to your life partner about his feelings too as he has them as well. Togetherness, in itself, can be therapeutic.

Chapter 6

The World of Infertility in the Pandemic

When it rains, it pours! As if a shocking infertility diagnosis is not enough, patients are grappling with fear and uncertainty due to the pandemic. No one saw this coming. The WHO, ASRM, infertility clinics, and patients did not know how to navigate the quest to conception with such an invisible and destructive virus infamously known as Covid-19.

The pandemic forced infertility clinics to shut down in many areas at the during the pandemic. Clinics abruptly halted treatments, and many patients had their treatment canceled mid-cycle. Many patients also lost their jobs; hence their healthcare coverage and income. The chaos that suddenly hit the globe and specifically the world of infertility was one we will not forget. We will never know how many women would have conceived and been on their way to having their babies.

Yet, the data is still very fluid, and the threat to pregnancies and the health of babies born to COVID-19 mother is not adequately known. This uncertainty drives a silent fear in parents-to-be, whether by natural conception or infertility treatments.

One of my patients, an emergency department (ED) intern, became pregnant in February 2020 for the first time after two failed IVF attempts. She then miscarried at 7 weeks, right at the onset of the pandemic. She stated that she will never know if she lost her baby because of COVID-19. There is limited information on how COVID-19 affects the fetus or how it will affect the babies conceived in this pandemic.

As an infertility nurse who works in Utilization Management (UM) for major insurance companies that provide infertility coverage, I have seen the torrents of treatments that flow in for prior authorization. These include new authorization requests and re-authorization of treatments that were abruptly halted.

While the race to having a baby becomes more urgent, the stress mounts; added to this is the layer of uncertainty. According to the CDC, ASRM, and state guidelines, patients must get a COVID test 72 hours before egg retrieval or embryo transfer. If the test comes back positive, the cycle is canceled.

Consider the waste of the effects of expensive fertility drugs – thousands of dollars which may not be fully covered by insurance, the eggs which would not be fertilized, and the babies who will not be born.

Another tragedy is the loss of both income and insurance benefits due to unemployment. I have counseled patients whose stress levels have increased in desperation to get their treatment started due to the risk of losing their jobs and insurance coverage.

There is the "medically necessary" infertility treatment to freeze eggs, sperm, or embryo freezing for men and women of childbearing age who are newly diagnosed with cancer. Cancer treatment, such as surgery, chemotherapy, and radiation threaten fertility. Hence childbearing age patients who desire to have children must quickly undergo this fertility treatment before cancer treatment. Fertility specialists and their staff across the country must carefully prioritize treatments for this population while staying within the CDC, ASRM, and state guidelines to prevent the spread of COVID-19. Dr. Eric Forman from the prestigious Columbia University recorded on YouTube the multi-factorial layers of concerns and evolving RE medicine practices in the pandemic (Forman, 2020).

The stress mounts. A survey conducted by a panel of doctors at Columbia University Fertility Center concluded that "given the severity of the COVID-19 pandemic, the physical, financial, and emotional impact of this unprecedented threat cannot be underestimated in our fertility patients" (Turocy, 2020.)

Steps that providers have taken to curb the effects of this pandemic are:

- limit staff in the facility.
- have patients wait in their cars until it's their turn to come into the clinic.
- teleconference instead of in-person consultations to determine the type of infertility treatments to be performed.

These steps have consequences. For example, patients who postponed treatment until lost jobs due to the pandemic. With loss of both income and coverage, the stressors increase. I heard from a couple of patients who rushed to beat the shut-down and started treatment cycles only to face cancellation because the patients contracted COVID-19 during treatment. This has been devastating. They were forced to get off the costly medications and quarantine.

It became difficult to advise patients and providers on how to most effectively proceed except to pay attention to the fluid data, abide by the limited scope of practice, follow the ever- changing CDC and state guidelines, and wait to see how it all pans out.

Clinics started to open in the summer, and the floodgates have swung wide open. The world of infertility became extremely busy, including specialty pharmacies. COVID surges affect the ability of patients to get treatment. The consequences and stressors continue to mount.

Up to this point, I've shared a lot of data and medical concepts. Now it is time to meet the people behind the data.

Part Two

IT HAPPENED TO ME: PATIENTS' STORIES

Part Two contains the emotional, multi-layered, stress-provoking, and thrilling memoirs of several patients and their nurse as they take you down this path and into their worlds of infertility.

In-vitro fertilization (IVF) plus assisted reproductive technology (ART) and adoption were shrouded in much secrecy not so long ago but are more openly discussed as women feel compelled and empowered to share their joys of fulfillment. As they do so, they help to strengthen other women who feel lost. Still, IVF using donor eggs, donor sperm, and donor embryos continues to be a well-kept secret.

Chapter 7

Margaret Davies

Though the journey may be rugged and paved with much pain and disappointment, embrace it, because you must aim for the finish line, as therein lies the purest of joys that await.

— Pamela G. Rasheed, MSN, RN

Author's note: As a fertility nurse, I had never met one person who did it all – IVF with autologous eggs (her eggs), donor eggs, husband's sperm, donor sperm, and adoption, until I met Margaret. She is the mother of five beautiful children and forever grateful for each one. Margaret was not my patient, but together as specialty nurses, we provide care and support to infertility patients throughout the USA. Here is her story.

When Pamela asked me to write my story, I was happy to share what I went through to help someone else. Pamela is a nurse who cares a great deal about what infertile people need to go through to achieve the greatest gift in life: children.

When I am writing something incredibly important, I first write in my mind, then on paper. Fortunately, and unfortunately, reliving my story stirred up memories that I thought I had put to bed. During this process, I needed to remind myself that I am a wonderful woman who has always been enough.

Infertility destroys a woman's self-esteem, and many marriages end in divorce because of infertility. Then it tears out your heart after you live through a pregnancy loss, and when you hear inappropriate comments, it turns your guts inside out. I lived through that – it is my story.

Every person in this world has a story to tell. Everyone has gone through some type of pain and hurt. But know this, the good Lord has given us tools to work through our pain; it is just the journey that is difficult. Then once we get through it, we pray we never experience that type of problem again. Yes, I am willing to stand in the storm if it will help another person to know that she (or he) is enough! You will make it through. Most importantly, whatever is meant to be will be.

Go on the journey if it is yours and use the tools along the way. Be open to options; be ready to use your voice, too; and know you do not have to be alone. There are many excellent support services available. There is hope. Muster up all your courage; be ready to accept whatever comes your way and go for it! In the end, it is all worth the journey. Know there is always a rainbow after the storm.

Getting Pregnant Would be Easy

I always thought it should be easy to conceive and have babies. Our bodies were meant to procreate. When I was growing up, no one knew what infertility was. When I grew up, no one talked about poor Aunt Margaret, at least not to her face, about why she did not have children. Why was she bitter and broken? No one asked Uncle George why he was always extra nice to his nieces and nephews. No one wanted to know because they, too, felt powerless to utter a word about what they know was supposed to happen naturally in life but did not.

Growing up, we all learned to believe that everyone was supposed to graduate high school and college, get a job, find that perfect someone, get married, and ultimately have children—until they found out they could not achieve the goal of having children. What was "wrong" with them?

I was 27 and very ready to start my family. I completed all the precursors with flying colors. I had a fantastic career as a nurse, and I was newly married and, hopefully, awaiting pregnancy. It did not happen.

Because I worked at a facility with a fertility clinic, I thought, "Why not check it out?" So, I did, only to find myself in the corner of the exam crying when the doctor told me I would need surgery. I was broken.

What are You Crying For?

The nurse said to me, "What are you crying for? It is not a big deal." Little did she know I wanted a big family, but now it hit me like a bolt of thunder, just dreading that I might not even be able to have one child. Later, when I worked with this nurse, I let her know how her words not only dismissed me but were a slap in the face of my self-esteem.

Words do matter; our pain does matter; and most importantly, we matter! It was a valuable lesson for me to learn as a woman and a nurse. I refuse to be labeled as a disease entity; I am a person who has a medical condition that required surgery. From that moment on, I worked hard at remembering that fact for myself and my patients who are dealing with infertility.

Surgery 1990

In early May of 1990, I had surgery. My husband could not be with me, so I asked my parents to help me. This was extremely hard for me. I was ashamed and scared. They were older and did not understand what infertility meant. I had seven brothers and sisters. My parents came from big families.

My pain was so great; my inner voice could not believe it, let alone utter it. I would need surgery before I could even think of becoming pregnant. My folks had to drive 30 miles plus to assist me, and that meant more to me than anyone would ever know. My folks came to get me from the hospital, take me home, and bought me groceries. Their support was priceless.

When they said goodbye, I remember hugging my dad, not knowing I would never see him again. Two weeks after my surgery, my dad unexpectedly died. He would never meet his grandchildren if there were any. My grief increased exponentially. He was my rock and the person I admired most in this world. He was a creative, hardworking farmer, a man of integrity who taught me to believe things will work out. Thank God for great parents who know how to demonstrate strength and courage when it feels hopeless. They were God's gift to me.

Don't Tell Anyone

After my surgery, I needed to wait several months before I could start treatment. It was September 1990, and I would need in-vitro fertilization (IVF), a "Hope" cycle. Back then, a Hope cycle was very much like intrauterine insemination (IUI), with minimal medication. Still, we did the intramuscular injections with long needles into the hip, just not as much. Then they would retrieve the eggs out of my ovaries and inseminate them with my husband's semen. We also only used minimal sedation for egg retrievals. I was wide awake. My doctor was very gentle and genuinely kind.

The hardest part is I had to go through this procedure alone. My husband blamed me, and the doctor told me not to tell anyone because they would not understand what I was doing. Of course not! Who would understand my baby would have to be made in a test tube, and it would cost me over $20,000?

Money aside, the time, the shame, the blame, and the need for secrecy only added to the sense of despair and uncertainty. Additionally, there were no resources or advocates to help women like me cope with these procedures' non-medical aspects. At that time, we did not even know all the things that would need to be done to achieve pregnancy.

To mention one, I needed to self-administer intramuscular injections at an exact time twice a day. I had to give them to myself, in front of a long-length mirror, so I did not hit a nerve.

A Second Job to Pay for Eggs

I only recruited three follicles; the financial cost would be the same for the IVF services, whether I recruited one egg or twenty. Insurance did not pay for any of it. Sadly, I did not get pregnant. I needed to try again and to find more money to try again. I took on another job to pay the bills. I was working full-time as a hospice nurse, but now I added a part-time shift at the clinic where I was doing my IVF treatment. I saved enough money for round two.

The second cycle yielded many eggs – twenty-eggs, whoo hoo! My excitement was short-lived. Adding sudden grief and uncertainty, while I was having my egg retrieval, the doctor let me know that they could not use my husband's sperm because his sample had white blood cells, an indication of an infection or a contaminant. I needed to decide on a sperm donor right then and there. What a nightmare.

To add to the grief, just days later, the staff told me I only had six embryos on day three. We also had decided to do day-three biopsy for preimplantation genetic testing/screening (PGS), a new concept for women of advanced maternal age. I was just 34 and labeled as "advanced" maternal age. I would never have imagined that when life was supposed to be in full swing, I was already on the road downhill.

Because of PGS, I could not do a fresh embryo transfer but needed to wait for the test results that would determine which embryo was normal – that would be transferred back to my uterus, increasing my chance of pregnancy. Of course, this would need to be done later as a "frozen embryo transfer (FET). The FET cycle resulted in a chemical pregnancy. A "chemical" pregnancy?—was I pregnant or not? What happened? How could God be so cruel, to give me hope and then take it away? Never in my life did I feel more like a failure than I did during those years: the tears, the disappointments, the despair, the brokenness, and the fear of being barren. The harder I worked, the more desperate I became.

Shredding Marriage and a Third Job

This process seriously damaged my marriage, with the distance, the pressure of dealing with the finances, then more blame. Self-blame, finger-pointing, and shame ripped the beautiful fragment of my once-happy marriage to shreds I could not recognize. I felt alone.

Depleted of money, I needed to take a third job if I wanted to continue my journey to having a child.

I had an incredible offer to start teaching certified nurse's aides' class in the evening. This was an excellent opportunity to make an impact on nursing. Although I was broken over the failure to have a baby at this point, I was thrilled to help others to learn how to provide care and to understand the concept of empathy better. Not only did I need the resources, but I also wanted to make a difference to other members of the nursing profession.

By the grace of God, one of my coworkers was a woman who had gone through IVF a year before; it worked. She gave me hope, and she gave me support, unbeknownst to her. It must have been divine intervention that she was positioned in my path at this stage in my journey for this purpose. And for the first time, I felt, just maybe I could find success. So, I decided I would try again.

A Son – At Last

A little over a month later, I did a frozen embryo transfer of three embryos. We did it; it was worth the wait. But shortly into the second trimester, I learned I had lost one of my twins. I experienced fear, uncertainty, and devastation all over again. Then my little baby boy was born at 32 weeks. Weighing less than one pound, he was a fighter; he was a miracle. He was just like his grandfather, with whom he shares his name.

Then just six days after his miraculous entry into the world, still in the neonatal care unit (NICU), my son extubated himself, and at one point, we thought we would lose him. He suffered seizures and was diagnosed with Tourette's at the age of three.

Today, I have an incredible 29-year-old who is a true gift to this world, completing his Masters in Anthropology on his way to his doctorate. My one-pound preemie, my fighter baby defying all odd—only by God's grace and mercy.

End of Marriage

After my beautiful son was born, my marriage failed. It was too much for my husband. He could not go on. So, I went it alone—I tried to understand during this incredibly sad and painful time in my life. I reminded myself daily that I had the most precious bundle of joy, a precious gift from God. "A true miracle", as the nurses in the Neonatal Intensive Care Unit used to say.

I was finally allowed to take my son home when he was barely five pounds. Blessed kid (some may say "poor kid"), he could not breastfeed, he was smaller than my breast. My babysitter criticized me because I did not feed him properly. I could not even be a good mother, the one thing I had dreamed of being since I was eight years old. My self-esteem was still being challenged, but I kept on keeping on – I had a reason for this, my five-pound bundle of pure joy.

Search for Egg Donor

How could I possibly have more? Yet I still had frozen embryos to transfer. I always wanted more children. I wanted a big family, so at the age of 36, I headed back to transfer my frozen embryos. Two negative pregnancy tests later, my new doctor told me if I wanted to get pregnant again, my best chance was to get an egg donor.

To a nurse, it made sense. To a woman who came from a large family, it was nonsense—I was shocked. Yet I wanted children. I spoke to the clinic psychologist, an incredibly supportive woman who had also undergone IVF treatment. Yes, I would go forward. So, I went in search of an egg donor.

This concept was still new, and donors were not readily available, in part because of the need for confidentiality and anonymity. During this process, I also began thinking about adoption and started a file that sat on my dresser. However, I accumulated the money. I found an egg donor, and I went through another embryo transfer. When I got pregnant, I was elated. My son would have a sibling - my little boy made a small paper bed so a baby would come. But I miscarried again.

I found out after the loss that I had a uterine polyp. Still to this day, I am saddened and shocked that the doctor did not do a uterine evaluation before we did an embryo transfer. I was a nurse; why did I not know to ask? Then I think, maybe, my little one was not meant to be. It was a small soul, just needing a way home. I pray for my babies who left before I could meet them, and I know they are in God's arms.

Another surgery and two more embryo transfer cycles later, I still could not achieve pregnancy. I was devastated yet again. What could I do? The sadness was overwhelming, but my journey continued.

"My Husband Just Looks at Me, and I Get Pregnant"

During this time, I started teaching children's karate classes with my then 3-year-old son. One evening during my class, the parents in the dance studio started to talk about having kids. Here I stood to hear more hurtful words. The dance mothers in the school hallway were carelessly talking about how their "husbands just had to look at them, and they would get pregnant."

One woman was so very careless with her words as they chatted about monitoring ovulations to become pregnant. She blurted out, "Who needs all this witchcraft and voodoo?" I felt so hurt, to dream so big and to feel so small. What more could I do? Was it time to let go of my dream? Be satisfied with one child? After all, I was single; my son was having challenges. Was it time to give up on my dreams and desire to have even one more child?

New Love

Then came a gift - perfectly timed by God, my creator. I met an incredible man who thought my son and I were perfect, more than I could have ever dreamed of, more than I would have ever expected. Interestingly, we had met years before by phone when we worked in hospice. I would never have thought one day I would marry this special man. We would build a beautiful life together.

A New Pregnancy

My husband wanted more children as much as I did. Out of the blue, at 43, I became pregnant. What a wonderful way to unite our family— a natural pregnancy. I miscarried again. My husband was supportive.

Throughout the years, I had been collecting information about adoption. Was it time to take a step further? I pondered this on my way to have my pregnancy test repeated, with all the money gone, my dreams dashed.

Foster Care

But there sat Tommy's face on my dresser. We decided to consider foster care, a chance to build our family, and help the community. Then one day, into our life came our two middle boys, three and five years old, hurt, scared, and sad. We met at McDonalds. When I picked up the youngest, he clung to his milk carton and chocolate chip cookies, saying, "Mine." My heart melted like butter, and I was hooked.

Oh, yes, they challenged us every day of our life; however, we would never have changed the gift we were given. Our two boys taught us that life is precious. Both have chosen to follow their own dreams of becoming better today than they would have otherwise been. We know we gave them that opportunity, and we will be forever grateful to their dad, who had to let them go to make them ours.

Adoption

The Bible says, "Blessed is he (or she) whose quiver is full" (Psalm 127:5). Two years later, a friend and neighbor approached us, asking if we would adopt their baby due in one month. She was born on a Wednesday; my husband was able to be at her birth. We were expected to pick her up at 5 PM on Friday. We waited; we were ready. The boys were prepared for a real miracle. I would have my baby girl. Then the call came at 9:00 AM on Friday, "The mother had changed her mind." My heart was shattered. I can only tell you that the pain of those words ripped out my heart. Thank God for my coworkers and the doctor for who I worked. They gave me the love to survive the day.

At 5:00 PM, the call came, "Come get her; she is yours." In 2020, my beautiful daughter graduated from high school and has a heart filled with love. Never in this world would I have imagined that I would build my family in this unique way. I love each of my children with my whole heart and would not change the unique paths they followed to come to us.

It was "a full circle." It was never what I would have thought or understood would be my life. Traditionally, this is not how families become families; yet I changed *my* story. I made my beautiful family whole, and I did it my way.

Today the world of infertility, adoption, and gestational surrogacy is more available. It is no longer a secret or something shameful. However, it is still very costly, and it still tears away at your self-esteem. It can rip marriages apart, or it can be a foundation of courage and love beyond what you could imagine. I learned that nothing is ever the way we want it to be or the way we think it is supposed to be. If we can ask, dream, and envision, then we need to garner all our strength and faith, then move forward.

In closing, I admonish you. Believe in yourself and your future. Do not negate the possibilities. Above all, never give up hope. Life is a journey filled with many obstacles; do not let them get in your way. Now I pray for grandbabies to wrap my arms around and tell them the stories of their parents, my children who came to me in incredibly special and unique ways.

This is my story of love, written by a wonderful woman, loving wife, and mother filled with gratitude as a patient and nurse. Journey on, and never be afraid to search for a satisfying end to your story.

"Creating a family in this turbulent world is an act of faith, a wager that against all odds there will be a future, that the heart can triumph against all adversities and even against the grinding wheel of time.

— **Dean Koontz**

Chapter 8

Melissa and Josh Petrella

Don't expect everyone to understand your journey, especially if they have never had to walk your path.

— **Reproductive Care Center**

I come from a big family. Writing my story brought back the uncomfortable memories of continually preparing for baby showers of my friends and families when I was secretly struggling with conceiving. At times it seems like every year, my family was celebrating a baby shower and children's birthday parties, but I had no idea that I would ever have trouble having children of my own.

Being so Careful – for What?

It was naïve of me to think I had done everything right with college, career, and settling down with the man I had been dating since my second year of college. Therefore, having a baby would be as easy. On the other hand, Josh was the youngest of four siblings and expecting a nephew in the fall. Josh did not even think of the word "infertility," but then it suddenly became a word written all over our very existence. I was even incredibly careful to use birth control for one year after our much-awaited wedding and honeymoon. As I liked to call it, this one-year honeymoon was filled with trips and birth control pills. But to my shock, I discovered that getting pregnant was not a walk in the park.

I eventually turned to the Internet, and what I read gave me a frightening awakening. I wondered, "Is it possible I have an infertility issue?" I couldn't bring myself to discuss this matter with Josh; after all, he was too excited about the impending arrival of his sister's third baby, another little tyke to spoil, he would say.

"When Will You Be Next?"

I began to feel dread at the thought of attending my sister-in-law's baby shower because I knew I might not be able to hide my feelings. Lately, my mother-in-law had been making comments about Josh not giving her grandkids. I sat in her living room, surrounded with laughter and chatter and piles of baby clothes and toys. Then I heard comments suggesting that I would next add to the family's growth into which I married.

But at thirty-four years old, I had not conceived over the last eight months of trying. As our second wedding anniversary approached, I found the courage to talk to Josh about my potential fear, which he brushed off with the notion that I was overthinking. All I needed to do was focus on the fertile period of my menstrual cycle. He brazenly pointed out that I should start checking for the accurate time of my cycle to become pregnant.

But after several months of over-the-counter ovulation predictor kits (OPK) and basal body (BBT) temperature checks, I remembered my conversation with Connie, my college roommate, who mentioned a while back about monitoring her fertility window with OPK. I decided it was time to make an appointment with my gynecologist (GYN). At that appointment, Dr. Sanders checked my AMH (Anti-Mullerian hormone) level that predicts ovarian reserve. It indicated that the level was 1.09 ng/ml.

Although Dr. Sanders said it was normal, she also said it was on the lower end of normal for a woman of thirty-four. She referred me to an infertility specialist and encouraged me to take Josh to this critical appointment. After a repeated AMH and FSH (follicular stimulating hormone), hysterosalpingogram (HSG) – a study of the fallopian tubes to rule out the blockage, and a semen analysis for Josh, we scheduled a follow-up appointment to review test results and come up with a plan.

I could not sleep for several nights before the follow-up appointment. Josh spent more hours at work and time hanging out at his brother's place. I gathered that it was his way of dealing with his anxiety.

What's Wrong?

At that crucial appointment, the physician defined our torrent of misfortunes. Not only did I have a "low egg reserve" (AMH of 0.99 ng/ml), but Josh had a "low sperm morphology" (normal shape of sperm). My HSG revealed a potential distal tubal block, which Dr. Sanders pointed out might be canalized (opened with another HSG procedure).

This was too much for me to absorb, while Josh just brushed it off again, saying that "we need to keep trying on our own." After several more months of trying for one chance of one lucky sperm to meet one lucky egg in the only open fallopian tube, the stress was like taking a once-a-lifetime test with great odds of failing.

The Stress Mounts

Coupled with Josh's resistance to clinical interventions Dr. Sanders advised, I began to think I was a failure. Josh's emotional withdrawal brought more despair and stress to the equation. Sex was no longer fun or enjoyable but rather mechanical only to "engineer a family," and it seemed that I was alone. Time began to pass so slowly – and yet so quickly.

On our third anniversary, I managed to snag a promise from Josh that we would proceed with intrauterine insemination (IUI). As the doctor explained it, this was a procedure to inseminate me with a laboratory-prepared sample of Josh's sperm at the time of my ovulation, which would be predicted by ultrasound and blood tests monitored by Dr. Sanders. Three attempts of failed IUIs and potentially a lower AMH and sperm morphology continued to drain me emotionally and psychologically.

At the same time, we heard that another one of Josh's sisters and his brother's wife were both pregnant again, each with their second child. I wanted to crawl into a dark hole and stay there rather than to endure yet more baby showers and comments of "What are you waiting for? The honeymoon is long over." Little did anyone know that we were dealing with male and female infertility, something we both wanted to keep private.

Eventually, we learned that in-vitro fertilization (IVF) was our best option. How did we get here? After years of being extremely careful in preventing pregnancy with birth control pills and condoms, how could this possibly be? Would our health insurance cover these procedures? Would we need to borrow money— and if so, from whom? We pledged secrecy; our families and friends must never know that we were infertile. As a teacher with the New York City public schools, I couldn't get much coverage under Emblem Health Group Health Insurance. We added money worries to the mix. We both had responsible jobs, but our rent and other lifestyle needs ate up most of our combined income.

Who could we talk to? We couldn't talk to each other for fear that I would start to cry, and Josh would leave to "clear his head." Gloom set in; I could only think that we needed one attempt at IVF cycle, and we would be all set – we would have a baby. It was worth the thought, but Josh didn't want to take out a personal loan for IVF, and I didn't want to explain to my family why we couldn't have a child the natural way. Now looking back, we saw how much ego and pride came into play, in addition to fear of marital discord and childlessness.

IVF Starts

Our first IVF was quite stressful. Who expects a layperson, a second graders teacher, to know how to mix and administer Gonal-f and Menopur, then Certrotide and Novarel later in the cycle? How was I supposed to go for morning monitoring and get to the front of the class by 8:30 AM? How much I would have rather crawled into that dark hole in my imagination and stayed there forever or woken up to realize it was just a nightmare.

We decided to start the IVF cycle at the end of the school year in June and hopefully be pregnant by September 5. The summer was an emotional seesaw. I could not relax on the beach in a bikini because I was bloated. My infertility nurse told me swimming in the ocean was not an option. The day of my egg retrieval could not come and go quickly enough. I remember feeling like several days went by while I was in the recovery room. I was groggy but suddenly delighted to hear that the physician retrieved 12 eggs – I began to cry. I hoped that this would result in my family of three to four children.

This hope was truly short-lived and deflated by the next day. Dr. Sanders called to report that only 5 of the 12 eggs were fertilized. As she explained the potential drop-off rate over the phone, I felt nauseous and alone. Josh was at work. Dr. Sanders explained that this might be due to poor sperm morphology. She further explained a potential reduction in embryos over the next three to five days and that we might end with two or fewer embryos; there was no guarantee. The room began to spin.

Yes, Dr. Sanders defined all these possibilities earlier to manage our expectations, but I selectively ignored them because I didn't want to contemplate them. I dreaded failing a once-in-a-lifetime test again.

By nightfall, I was bloated and uncomfortable – insomnia caused me to toss and turn in discomfort as I wept. I called the emergency on-call nurse, who answered immediately and offered support. Ovarian hyperstimulation was a new terror, and all this while Josh appeared to be emotionally distant.

New grief hit me. What was happening to my relationship and friendship with my husband? This was not something I wanted to face because if I focused on positive thoughts as the nurse encouraged, I might well get pregnant, and my marriage would be just fine.

As Dr. Sanders predicted, there were two "good" quality embryos at the end of the cycle. She advised us to have a single embryo transfer to reduce the risk of multiple babies and complications such as early delivery, NICU time, and other issues. We agreed. We were excited; there was a light at the end of this long and dreary tunnel.

Embryo Transfer

The embryo transfer procedure just six days after the egg retrieval was smooth, and despite mild ovarian hyperstimulation, I felt optimistic. I determined to get enough rest while my precious embryo swam around and found a spot on my uterus wall to implant. The staff preserved one embryo for a later pregnancy.

But day ten after embryo transfer, I started to bleed like a period. I was devastated. After thousands of dollars, many nights of uncomfortable self-injections, emotional roller coasters, I failed to get pregnant. I was in shock. The nurse requested that I head into the clinic for a blood test. She explained that sometimes the bleeding might mean that the embryo didn't implant; it implanted, and I had a biochemical reaction, or I was pregnant. I needed a test to find out.

My neighbor Nancy dropped by as I was processing this agony, and after one look at me, she became concerned. I began to cry hysterically and told her half the story. She did not question further but offered to drive me to the subway just a few blocks away to the appointment.

My insides turned upside down when I heard the words, "I am so sorry, but your pregnancy test is negative. You need to take a break and allow your ovaries to get back to baseline before attempting another IVF cycle" said the second-year fellow, Dr. Angelina Ross.

"What do you mean?" I felt chills and despair, "I cannot do this when school reopens!" I wept uncontrollably. Josh walked over to attempt a comforting gesture but withdrew. He was not sure I would accept it; after all, he was the reason for "poor fertilization." I was angry at him, and he knew it.

The Student Becomes the Mentor

I grieved and felt alone. It soon became September, and the school reopened. By chance, a new second-grade teacher, Lauren, came on, and I was her mentor. As we worked together, I learned that she went through two IVF cycles and was again pregnant with her second child after three failed embryos, two miscarriages at eight and ten weeks, and five years of infertility. She gave me hope.

Lauren encouraged me to see an acupuncturist and to do mindful meditations. She also told me how she coped with stressors in her marriage, and she had continued to use the mindful app to meditate daily after successfully delivering her son two years before. She also encouraged me to find someone in my circle who I trusted to talk to about my fears. These methods helped her. Lauren said these interventions gave her an outlet. I thought that God sent this teacher my way. If not, I would not have known how to continue. Lauren became that friend I trusted, and she was so incredibly supportive.

I went back to Dr. Sanders and discussed a frozen embryo transfer of the one remaining embryo. Whether Josh was supportive or not, I was going for it. I met with Miss Leoung for acupuncture according to the schedule recommended.

The FET cycle was not as expensive or intensive as IVF. As I learned, the embryos are already available and frozen from the IVF cycle. Now the uterus needs to be prepped with minimal medications to be receptive to the embryo. Though I dreaded failure, I found the nightly meditation helped me relax and think more positively. Nurse Pam, who had always been supportive and never judgmental, was happy to hear that I was getting acupuncture, something she had encouraged before. At my FET procedure, she squeezed my hand and said, "Melissa, I think that all the stars are lined up." From the way she saw it, Lauren came to me to help me.

The Pilgrim's Promise

As I waited for 15 minutes after my embryo transfer, Pam told me about the "Pilgrim's Progress," a story of how people show up in our lives at different stages to help with what we need at those stages. I took that thought home with me: "The stars are lined up." My pregnancy test was positive for the first time, and except for one first trimester scare of unexplained bleeding, we had a healthy bouncing baby boy, Andrew.

What I went through and how useless I felt as a barren woman is just a dark memory tucked away in history. My baby changed my life. As a NYC teacher, my health plan GHI covers three IVF cycles and three FET cycles, which my diagnosis qualifies me for, and soon we will embark on having a sibling for our son.

The pain, the grief, the fear, and the financial dread are real. And yes, you may feel lonely and alone in your relationship. Find outlets for these demons. Do not let them stay in your space. You may not trust anyone to share your fear or secret of infertility but own your story and embrace the challenges that come with it.

If there is a will, trust God, and He will make a way. He will also send someone to help, like in Pilgrim's Progress. I am complete – I am a mother.

Even miracles take a little time.
—Cinderella's Fairy Godmother

CHAPTER 9

CASANDRA AND DANIEL WILLIAMS

Give all your worries and cares to God, for he cares about you.
— 1 PETER 5:7 NLT

I have a disease called endometriosis, identified at the age of 31-years-old. When I received the diagnosis, I was shocked to know I might not have children. I do not think it hit me until we began to try in-vitro fertilization treatments. Our very first try using my own eggs was a nightmare. I conceived but experienced a miscarriage and almost ended up dying while undergoing a dilatation and curettage (D&C) procedure in the operating room (OR).

Facing the Realities

After that traumatic event, my husband and I decided to stop trying for a couple of years. We were just too scared. However, our dream of having a family did not stop. After moving from New York to New Jersey, we sought help from another reproductive endocrinologist. We were hopeful we might be successful, given that I at least had gotten pregnant before. Again, our hope was dashed when the next two IVF cycles were also unsuccessful. We stopped because my health insurance did not cover infertility treatment, such as IVF, and we could not afford to pay privately.

This is when the emotional and psychological devastation started to become real, and the awareness finally began to sink in that having children might not be in our future. We considered adoption, but then again, it was a financial dilemma. We were not financially ready.

After a while, a good girlfriend of mine who knew of my plight and saw my despondency suggested using a surrogate in India. In this case, I would still be able to have a baby with my own eggs but have a borrowed uterus to carry my baby to term. We knew of another couple who went through with this plan. Unfortunately, they went to India, but surrogacy did not work for them either; hence we threw that option out as well.

I started to think, "What else is there to do with my life?" I fulfilled all my goals, including a career as a registered nurse and married a wonderful man, except for having my children and knowing what's it's like to be a mom. What was I going to do with the rest of my life? I was now without purpose. I just did not know what was left to do.

Everyone around me had children. Not for a moment did I wish this dreadful plight on my worst enemy. I was grateful for the unstoppable support I had. Some of my close girlfriends knew what I was going through. I did not mind going to baby showers because I was always happy for others, but I kept longing to have a baby. My husband wanted a child, and he would do practically anything to have a child too. I saw the stress he was going through. And I knew he was worried about me also.

One More Try

We then decided to try one more time. I took a year off from trying, but I could not stop bleeding from the medications I was taking for the in-vitro. I went back to my original reproductive endocrinologist. The physician explained I had to have surgery again before starting IVF. This seemed like a never-ending painful journey, but I continued to hold fast to my idea of having my baby one day. This was just the beginning of yet another step on this journey.

After the surgery, the physician told me I would not need a surrogate; I would be able to carry a pregnancy. However, I would need an egg donor because my egg reserve was depleted due to the endometriosis and the repeated surgeries. More questions fluttered in my head. It was a lot to comprehend. And to add to all this, we were anxious about the financial toll it would take on us.

My friends and family volunteered to donate their eggs, but due to scheduling conflicts and age factors, having one of them donate was impossible. I finally started to think that maybe I was not meant to have children; however, it didn't mean I couldn't be a mother to someone – I could explore adoption.

"What Would God Think?"

I began to question my Catholic faith. "What would God think? Was I forcing the hand of God? Should I have children this way? Would I be punished? Having to use someone else's eggs to give me a baby is not natural," I said to myself. So many questions and nagging thoughts flooded my mind. After all the fretting emotionally, spiritually, and psychologically, I eventually began to let go and let God take over. I was at the end of my ability to continue to try. My faith took over, and I finally released this desire to my creator - GOD. That is when things began to take on a new perspective and energy.

My husband and I decided to move forward with donor IVF. There was only one problem: money. We planned to solve that problem by taking out a loan on our 401k. However, we were short on time to get this done. My parents were no longer living. My mother-in-law knew of our struggles, but she never pressured us or ever asked us when we were going to give her grandchildren. (My husband is her only child.) As a result, I have so much respect for her up to this day. Knowing that she must want grandkids and experiencing her silent kindness became an added reason to continue trying. She became my second mother. She treats me as if I were the daughter she always wanted. I thank God for her every day.

An Unexpected Sale

My mother-in-law sold her condominium just to give us the money we needed to proceed. (She claimed that she was going to sell it anyway.) After she gave us the money, she never asked any questions. We started filling out the paperwork, and it was a go. The fertility center found us a donor.

My conversations with God began to get simpler. I told God, "You got this, and I am letting go." I followed all the directions given to me clinically by my doctor and my nurse and spiritually by what I felt inside my inner being. After I did what I needed to do, I let go and let God do what He alone can do: miracles.

Let God, Let Go

I stopped thinking about my efforts to get pregnant. Even when they took my blood to check to see if I was pregnant, I allowed myself to let go. "The levels are rising, and they are rising appropriately," said my nurse, and I did not think or worry how it would all end. I was pregnant, drained of worrying, and ready to let God do the rest.

When I went in for my first ultrasound, and the doctor pointed out my baby's heartbeat, was THE moment I knew it was real. This worked. I was pregnant. I had never heard a baby's heartbeat before. It was incredible. I heard life.

How Many Heartbeats?

The second ultrasound was a shocker: there were two babies' heartbeats. Yes, twins. My conversations with God went like this: "Thank you, God, for blessing me with these gifts; I just want these babies to be healthy. Give me the strength to carry these beautiful gifts you have given me. I do not care if there are two boys or two girls, or one boy and one girl…I just want them to be healthy."

My prayers were answered. I was blessed with double for my trouble. God is good all the time. He gave us two beautiful, healthy bundles of ultimate bliss and joy – a boy and a girl, Christian and Isabella.

My life is fulfilled and has never been the same. The twins are five years old. They have all the energy in the world, and they have turned my world right-side-up. I promise to take care of them and enjoy them for the rest of my life. What is crazy is that I cannot remember what I was doing or what my life was before these little bundles of joy came along.

> *Don't confuse your path with your destination. Just because it's stormy now doesn't mean that you aren't headed for the sunshine.*
>
> **—Smart Fertility Choices**

Chapter 10

Jill and Jack Hudson

Impossible is just a word thrown around by small men who find it easier to live in the world they've been given than to explore the power they have to change it. Impossible is not a fact. It is an opinion. Impossible is potential. Impossible is temporary. Impossible is nothing.

— Muhammad Ali

The author of this book, Pamela Rasheed, was one of the people who helped successfully manage my IVF journey. I hope my story will serve as inspiration for prospective parents who choose to have children this way. Pamela was the gentle nurse who held my hand at every step and guided me through the complicated process. She kept me disciplined and focused on my goals as a patient.

Under Pamela's guidance as Nurse Coordinator, I felt fully aware and informed about every aspect from the start to "graduation day," the day the fertility clinic released me to my OB-GYN at eight weeks pregnant. Pamela was part of the team who helped bring about not just one miracle baby, but two. She believes that aside from the scientific data in this book, the unique personal stories from her previous patients who have gone through the IVF journey will positively change the experiences of future IVF patients. I believe in her mission and trust her with my story.

At the age of fifty-two, I had my first IVF miracle baby. At the age of fifty-four, I had my second IVF miracle baby.

Choosing When to Get Pregnant

As I got older, and new scientific advancements in IVF became more socially mainstream, I saw the possibility that my biological clock would no longer determine my gestational future. IVF allowed me to make a conscious and responsible decision to conceive and eventually give birth again at a later and wiser age. I felt liberated by the possibility of expanding my family at any time and not be stigmatized or limited by society's opinion that I was simply "too old" to have children.

Nevertheless, this journey still required significant effort and dedication. Many critical factors affected my path to motherhood. I grappled with the commitment to start the journey, the absolute determination to complete the process, and the acceptance of only the highest standards from myself and the people involved, regardless of the outcome. IVF demanded a challenging intellectual and emotional investment. I had to reach through the depths of my experiences for strength to complete the process and to prepare for the unguaranteed outcomes. Every individual has a different source from which to find strength, and mine was what I learned from my mother.

All Sister Family

The day I was born, I was considered my mother's sixth failure to give my father a baby boy. I was born during a time when most people believed the woman determined the sex of the fetus. In the year 2020, I hope people know it is in fact, the man who determines the sex of the fetus.

Like most societies throughout history, the Asian society I was born into valued boys over girls. My mother suffered much criticism for giving birth consecutively to six baby girls. During my early childhood in Asia, boys were considered worthy of financial investments, education, and inheritance of real estate. Boys grew into leadership positions. Women who gave birth to boys received compliments, but women who did not got criticized.

As a result of this social discrimination against baby girls, my mother invested her love, time, and financial abilities to nurture my five sisters and me despite our sex. We were loved, educated, and valued. My mother taught us to cherish ourselves. As early in my childhood as I can recall, my mother raised me to believe societal traditions or restrictions did not predetermine my future.

Importance of Education

Schools were not free. Yet my mother made the rare investment of sending me to school. She truly believed that education was the greatest societal equalizer that would give me a chance to succeed. She said, "Education does not discriminate." She impressed upon me that education is the ladder to my potential, and desire is the seed to my dreams. My mother gave me the greatest gift, along with her love, when she encouraged me to attain my education, dream fearlessly, and dream big.

During my childhood in America, my mother used to tell me about her dreams. Her wistful smile was her acceptance that her dreams were daydreams due to her circumstances as a refugee. She lost everything in war and to Communists. Although I smiled back at my mother during these chats, I felt her sadness because her suffering was my suffering. My mother viewed her life in America as an existential survival without opportunity. Her only goal was to endure and help me fulfill my dreams because I was part of America and its future. I would live the American Dream.

The Gift

My mother burst with pride when I graduated from college. I immediately put my degree to work and got a job in the fashion industry. At twenty years old, I waited what seemed forever to be able to give my mother back some of her dreams. I remembered one of my mother's dreams was to own a fur jacket. Fashionable, elegant women in her time and culture wore fur coats during special social appearances. My mother was a minimalist and dreamed of a fur jacket.

With my first paycheck, I purchased a modest short rabbit fur jacket from a wholesale fur store in the fashion market.

It cost me a negotiated $99, my weekly salary. My mother did not care that it was rabbit fur and not mink or sable. When I surprised her with this gift on an ordinary day, a magnificent smile came to her face; we fulfilled both our dreams

I failed at fulfilling all my mother's dreams. My mother dreamed of visiting Paris since she had studied French. She died unexpectedly before I had a chance to make her Paris dream come true. This missed opportunity is my greatest regret—and a hard lesson learned. The pain of this failure taught me never to have daydreams, but true desires and dreams.

The Marathon Begins

At the age of forty-one, my thirty-year-old husband and I had one of those big dreams my mother encouraged. We confidently decided to have a baby with a clear understanding that our big dream of a family would take us on a quite untraditional gestational journey: IVF. My husband and I agreed that we could not take IVF lightly. It would not be a "magic bullet." Nor would it be a guaranteed success. It was clear to us that having a baby was about the baby and us. We were seeking an innocent life to come into our care as his or her parents.

My husband and I believed that our performance during our IVF journey was a statement about our worthiness to be parents. From the start to the outcome, this big dream of having a baby required our sincere and complete commitment to the IVF process. We were prepared for our IVF journey not to be a walk in the park, but a challenging marathon—an IVF Marathon.

As of 2019, *Runner's World* reported that less than .05 percent of the U.S. population has run a full marathon: 26.2 miles. At the age of forty, I dreamed of running a marathon. At the age of forty-one, I trained and ran the New York City Marathon for a charity. Though I did not foresee it as I crossed the finish lines of my marathons, I now realize the miles, sweat, pain, scrapes, and scars I earned from training and running the marathons helped give me the strength to endure the many mile markers as an IVF patient. I drew upon the strategies of discipline, perseverance, and faith as a marathon runner to manage the goals that were required to complete what I call "The IVF Marathon."

The Project Leader

When I ran marathons, I knew when and where to start: I started when the gun went off at the "Start" line. Once my husband and I decided to have a baby through IVF's help, the next questions were when and where do we start? Like mother like daughter, I believe that the difference between a dream and a daydream is execution. We could sit and talk about a dream, but it was merely a wistful daydream that would bring suffering to an unfulfilled soul without actual execution.

If we dared to have a dream, we needed to execute a plan to give our dream a chance to breathe life. Within a week of deciding to have a baby through IVF, I fired the "start" gun. Although my husband and I were a team in the IVF process, it was essential for us to elect a Project Leader for our home-front: me.

For a decade, I dedicated my mind, body, and lifestyle to my marathon commitments. This dedication was the reason for my successful training and finish. I ate, drank, and slept a marathon the second I entered the race. Each time I started training for a marathon, my goal was to cross the finish on race day. In my view, a successful marathon was a completed marathon regardless of time or placement; no matter what, I would cross the finish line.

This mindset was the only way that I found peace in the belief that I did my all to accomplish my goals, my dreams, including having a baby through IVF. Therefore, the purpose for our IVF Marathon was to finish no matter the outcome. I ate, drank, and slept our IVF process until the finish: "graduation day." As the Project Leader, it was up to me to set the standards for our IVF. The strategy was for us to find the best IVF doctors and clinic, be the best IVF patients, and finish with the knowledge that we did our best in our IVF journey to have a baby.

The Research Begins

I started the medical aspect of our IVF dream. The first call I made for my research into IVF was to a former trusted OB-GYN. She was always a caring doctor and person. She told me that "the odds were on my side" when I dared to attempt a successful pregnancy at the age of forty-six. I appreciated her surprisingly supportive words. Previously, others cruelly told me that "my time was up" for childbearing. Our dream back then was a "daydream."

"You Can Have a Baby in Your 50s"

Aside from the natural process, we did not honestly try to have a baby by all methods available. Once we were seriously committed to our IVF prospect, I spoke to her again. I believed that she would tell me if "my time was truly up." She also was incredibly supportive as a doctor and a woman. She referred us to a private clinic that she trusted and was successful with her patients. Our physician assured me that this innovative clinic had no issues with the challenge of my age. She confidently told me that she had patients in their fifties who had successfully had IVF and delivered healthy babies. For the first time, I realized our dream of a baby was a possibility. This hope was the result of the kind, supportive words from a caring professional and fellow woman.

Good advice is only useful if one takes it. At the recommendation of my former OB-GYN, I contacted the private IVF clinic she recommended. This was a great lead. The private clinic was eager to help us as a referral from my former OB-GYN. I realized that if there were one great IVF clinic willing to help us with our special IVF needs, there would be more. I interviewed a list of institutions that I believed would have the most innovative IVF methods.

As a believer in education, I narrowed my choices to include learning institutions in the West Coast and Northeast that were at the forefront of IVF science. My search narrowed further to New York City's exceptional learning institutions with IVF programs. One medical school clinic near my home stood out above all others as the most innovative with the most patient-friendly facility that I found in IVF medicine. Once I made my choice, I wasted no time. I updated my husband on my research results. With his agreement, I made an appointment that would later fulfill our dream to have a baby. I met with the IVF doctor who interviewed me as I assessed the clinic. It is essential to listen to one's instincts. My instincts said this was the right doctor, and this was the right clinic.

Committing to the Finish Line

For the doctor and the clinic to commit to us as patients, we had to commit to the process and the clinic. Many people leave their initial IVF appointment still in a daydream and not ready to go for the finish line. I let the doctor know that I was prepared for the commitment to finish, no matter the outcome.

This was also true the day I met Pamela. I had no doubt she was the gatekeeper to our IVF dream. I run with a faster and better runner when I want to improve my pace. In the IVF world, Pamela Rasheed was my quicker and better runner. She handed me two long lists of required physical and laboratory tests for my husband and me. She said that we could discuss the IVF process further when we completed the lists she gave me. I took a deep breath and got to work. In twenty days, we completed the tests. We passed the first mile marker of our IVF Marathon.

Financial Planning

When we dreamed of having our baby, we envisioned a precious little bundle of joy. However, our little bundle of joy costs money. Affordability was one of the first things that my husband and I discussed. Having a baby, whether through natural conception or IVF, costs money, *a lot* of money. It was not romantic to have finance first on the agenda when my husband and I decided on our dream to have a beautiful baby, but it was an essential strategic assessment. The reality was that IVF was expensive and a luxury.

One of my IVF strategies was to remove as many stressful issues as possible in preparation for the additional stress that we would have during our IVF process. We always hear that financial stress is an issue that destroys relationships. We did not start our IVF journey until we were ready and could pay for all the anticipated and unexpected expenses. We agreed that our dream of having a baby was worth our financial investment, no matter the outcome.

In addition to the cost of IVF, we prepared for the financial investment of raising our baby and providing him a life with unlimited opportunities. My husband and I were immigrants to the United States; we came from families with modest means. We knew what it was like to grow up economically underprivileged and agreed that we did not want our child to suffer the same socioeconomic struggles.

Passing the Tests

We were so happy with each phase we completed as we passed our physical examinations and laboratory tests. The healthcare team told us we could not proceed if we did not pass. It was critical to take these initial tests seriously.

They screened us (mostly me) to qualify us to be healthy IVF candidates with a good starting physical baseline for a successful outcome. My husband had one job for the clinic: to produce the sperm. As a woman, I had several tasks once the IVF cycle began. My uterus would be the home that would provide life to our fetus if the transplant was successful. This was the reason I made sure that I was a healthy candidate.

It was up to me to eat healthy foods. I made sure to keep up my fitness routine to maintain my optimal physical health. Under the guidance of the physician and Pamela, I had to be diligent with my medications and frequent monitoring appointments. This required absolute dedication to our IVF goals. As the Project Leader, I made sure to evaluate our commitment and provide updates and feedback at home and to the clinic every step of the way.

Overcoming Fear of Needles

We were thankful to the clinic team, who allowed us to pursue our desire for a baby. The doctors and Pamela were incredibly kind, helpful, and talented in their profession as Jack and I handled the administrative tasks exceptionally well. Although we had an immense fear of needles, we met the challenges of IVF practices that we did not expect, such as hormone shots. Pamela helped us face our fear of needles. She gave my husband lessons on injections until he was confident to do them. I had to believe he could competently inject me with a one-and-a-half-inch needle daily.

My husband was amazing once he graduated from Pamela's injection course. He is now a professional injection expert, but I will never be a happy injection recipient. Although my husband and I traveled through our IVF journey cohesively as a couple, there were issues that he could not understand because I was the only person living through many of the processes: the side effects of hormone medications, the multiple monitoring clinic visits, the numerous painful poking of needles, and so much emotional change.

I could not understand Jack's journey because he had different responsibilities and emotional challenges. He used to say that giving me shots hurt him more than it hurt me. This was the perfect example of our different experiences. We are not the type of people who use social media to publicize our issues. A book that honestly explained the experiences of IVF from a reputable, kind, and trustworthy professional written in simple language would have been a godsend for us.

Overall, I believe my husband and I had a very positive IVF experience. This was due to our commitment to each other, preparation for our goals, and respect for the professionals we chose to help us. We diligently did everything we were asked to do by the IVF team and met our clinic's financial requirements. We took every step and were unattached to expectations of a guaranteed outcome. Jack and I were able to do this because we had a contingency plan for multiple outcomes. Most importantly, we agreed to try with the understanding that IVF would not be a guaranteed success. If we tried IVF and had a negative result, we would accept our fate without regret and move forward.

Our contingency plan was adoption. Adoption is an extraordinary love: it is a love that an adopted parent chooses to have purely for the child, not because the child is in the parents' images. My husband and I agreed that we both could love a child regardless of whether he had our chromosomes. This made me love my husband more. Now that we are blessed with two children and know how important it is to love a child, we would welcome the opportunity to adopt a child. No child should be without love.

My incredible mother taught me remarkable things. These lessons gave me the courage to dream about fabulous journeys, as big, far, and wide as I could imagine. Since childhood, I have never lived a day without big goals. The bigger and the more spectacular my ambitions, the bigger my mother would smile when she heard about them.

The Yellow Lady Bug

I believe that if my mother knew I had a dream to have a baby at the age of fifty-two, she would have the biggest smile on her face and say, "That's my daughter!" This vision of my mother made my decision to try to have a baby at fifty-two through IVF, one of peaceful certainty. I believe that my mother was with us throughout the entirety of our IVF journey. When I took my pregnancy test for our first child through IVF, a rare yellow ladybug sat in my home with me until my husband returned home to release her back to nature.

As I left the clinic after taking a pregnancy test for our second child, a bird pooped on my new summer shoes. My parents believed it was good luck when a bird pooped on my father's new shirt.

I experienced the pressure of the "ticking clock" that women continue to endure about childbearing. When I faced my clock, I felt my value as a woman diminished because my time was up. I was once called "barren." My dream was to break that clock, not just to have a child for our family, but I believe it was to remove the imbalance that has plagued women since the beginning of human history. Men have chosen younger women as partners partly due to their biological ability to have children. IVF has extended a woman's ability to bear children. I believe that IVF has truly liberated women.

Chapter 11

Sadie Blackwell

I will go before you and make the crooked places straight; I will break in pieces the gates of bronze and cut the bars of iron. I will give you the treasures of darkness

And hidden riches of secret places that you may know that I, the LORD Who call you by your name, am the God of Israel.

– Isaiah **45:2-3**

No one ever told me how hard it was going to be. My quest to have a baby was passionate and relentless. As a new mother who wanted to devote all my time and energy to my baby, I never thought it would be anything short of bliss. But I came to realize how difficult it was. In reality, I've easily juggled work, the commute, the roles of a full-time employee, wife, and daughter of my elderly mother. When I added a baby to the equation, it meant more work, but I took it on with joy.

During my fertility journey, I did not focus on the difficulties of motherhood. It did not even occur to me that there would be challenges. I only focused on what it took to be successful at becoming a mother.

My daughter is a blessing, more than I expected, and I wouldn't have traded her for anything even if I had known it would be hard work.

Medical Barriers

The first step in my journey to have a child involved having several pints of blood drawn and tested. My highly skilled and renowned fertility specialist (over 30 years in the field) diagnosed me with Sjogren's, an autoimmune disease, and a stenosed cervix.

Although I was pregnant twice before I had my daughter, I could not retain the pregnancies. My doctor (Dr. Jeff Shapiro – a fictitious name) believed that the two times I became pregnant without IVF, I had spontaneous miscarriages due to Sjogren's. He said my body experienced the pregnancy as a foreign object invading my body and therefore fought to destroy it to keep me healthy.

Since my early twenties, I had struggled with year-round allergies that progressively got worse as the years passed on. At times I had sneezing, runny nose, irritated eyes, and an itchy and swollen face. I was keenly aware that this was my body's hypersensitive way of fending off something trying to assume residency in my body. I never thought that my immune system would work to betray me when it came to starting a family.

I wasn't convinced of the diagnosis at first. It seemed so farfetched and impossible. At least in my observations, millions of women have gone through worse diagnoses but could still conceive. Was it my body deceiving me, or were the specialists I was working with not familiar with my specific anatomy? Or, more likely yet, was my age a definite factor? I was 40 when my husband and I seriously started this quest to have a family. This was well beyond the childbearing years for women, even in today's modern times.

On the other hand, the stenosed cervix was a diagnosis that I immediately accepted. The fact that all of the practitioners I'd worked with spent 45 minutes or more attempting to transfer my embryo into my womb every single time was one indication of the diagnosis's accuracy. It was so challenging to enter my uterus that I was given anesthesia for five transfers, and it still had no impact on the length of time the procedure took. Incidentally, before one of the transfers, I was given a surgical cervix dilation. It made it slightly easier for the doctors to get their instruments in but still did not make a significant difference.

Once I awoke after a frozen egg transfer, the doctor at the facility, who did most of my transfers stated, "Yes, it was difficult to get in. You still have some embryos left." I knew what that meant. The physician destroyed my embryo in the process of trying to get into my cervix.

Besides feeling upset, I felt powerless about choosing a fertility facility and specialist who knew and understood my body. It may sound implausible to think doctors who work on women's anatomy are beginners, but in my experience, not all are experts in this area. I left that private fertility clinic and transferred to a top university hospital in NYC staffed with more doctors and more innovative options. I thought by doing so I would also have a fresh encounter and better outcome. Five years and six IVF transfers later, we were conducting the same process and procedures. It was abundantly clear to me that my providers needed a different approach. "But what" was the question.

Can We Try Something Different?

What I wished then was for one of the doctors to suggest trying something different. I finally had the guts to meet with Dr. Jeff Shapiro, my primary doctor at this top NYC facility, and petitioned him to consider another type of treatment. I was not sure there was another option, but I was willing to beg for it.

Looking back, I can say the doctor was a caring and progressive doctor who could not outright push his facility's boundaries. He arranged for me to work with another doctor in the field not affiliated with his facility. His unconventional treatment plan reportedly assisted in getting some women with autoimmune disorders pregnant. I'll call this older male doctor, Dr. David Shapiro. Coincidently, Dr. David Shapiro was trained in the same European country alongside Dr. Jeff Shapiro.

There's Hope

After reviewing my medical chart, Dr. David Shapiro was incredibly hopeful about our prospects of becoming parents. It was the first time in years that any doctor had given us even a glimmer of hope. I went through further testing and received new medications and treatments including Viagra and intralipid infusions that my medical insurance would not cover (because they were deemed experimental). All these efforts were the last attempts before my final IVF trial with the NYC facility. While Dr. David Shapiro made other recommendations for the frozen embryo transfer process, I received none of them due to my NYC facility's strict protocols. Unfortunately, no matter what new medications or solutions we tried, the same doctor at the NYC facility conducted the embryo transfer procedures. I did not conceive.

Could I Use an Egg Donor – Really?

I was shocked when I first learned about egg donors. Throughout this journey, I believed I would have two children who resembled our family in many ways, from the physical attributes to the emotional ones. These little humans would look and sound like my husband and me in every way. They would have my husband's soft and quiet way and my outspoken and sometimes reserved manner. Of course, God would grace us with healthy and happy children, I prayed. When I heard the words *egg donor*, I froze for at least five minutes as the doctor defined why I would be a good candidate for this program.

I was beyond devastated that trials with my eggs failed. Additionally, my ovarian reserve was quite low, and it would be challenging for me to conceive with my eggs.

My eggs didn't seem to be viable. I believed that having children was not the only role we were intended to fulfill on this planet. However, when I lost that option, I wondered if I would be a productive member of today's society without identifying as a mother. I pondered that seriously, especially considering my cultural background.

The expectations of my culture are that women bear children. I've heard people in my culture say that having *one* child is not sufficient. Producing more than a couple of children is preferable and more representative of womanhood. Though my parents were not always vocal on this point, I received subtle messages during my thirties about taking specific vitamins and not looking for the perfect situation to have a family.

So many questions came to me while I sat in that seat, thinking of the possibility of an egg donor for the first time. My head was spinning with feelings of blame, disappointment, and deep sadness. If I had to be completely transparent, I would say I was also furious at the facility and the different doctors I had worked with already. Why were they not able to deal with my unique structural difference properly? How is it that I had five perfect eggs, and they were all wasted throughout this process? Or at least that was how I felt. Even during that time, I couldn't quite express my distress. I recall mentioning it to my husband but not delving into how upset I was. He didn't understand the level of sadness and anger I felt.

Simmering Anger

When I look back on it now, I can see how my anger was slowly simmering. I felt betrayed by the individuals who took care of my fertility. My body let me down in a big way. I was also very angry with myself. Why had I waited all these years for marriage to have children? Why did I not start looking into preserving my eggs earlier? How could I keep working in a career where I saw parents and children regularly? Should I focus my energy and effort on helping to change the world in other ways that could support my urge to parent?

During the stages of IVF, I grappled with the realities of the treatment. I felt disbelief at what I had to go through. This shook me to the core. Was this my reality?

Making a Baby a Goal

For all my life, I considered a goal and worked hard towards it. Most times, with hard work, perseverance, and prayers, I achieved my aim. For example, getting through undergraduate and graduate school was a challenge because of a lack of funding and no family support. Nevertheless, I forced myself to graduate because I knew I had to have a specific skill set to find professional success for me. Hence, I braced up and made sacrifices. Landing work after acquiring the degrees was the same way.

Nothing has ever been easy for me. I am not complaining about that because I've learned to love the person I've become through some severe challenges. That is just how life is for some of us. This is not specific to only me. What I learned to understand about my pattern of struggle is that God always saw me to the other side. I landed on my feet despite the difficulties I had experienced. Nonetheless, in this case, I was not as convinced. Infertility was a hard blow; I was not expecting it.

I am not sure what snapped me out of my deep thought pattern that day in the doctor's office, but I eventually heard, "Would you like to set up an appointment to review the egg donor program?" My husband and I scheduled the appointment and met with a kind and caring doctor a month later. Dr. Brooke Rhinehart (fictitious name) was head of the egg donor program.

"Your Goal Is to Become a Parent"

As Dr. Rhinehart reviewed the program, I had tears in my eyes. She stopped and said words that put my heart at ease for the first time. "Your ultimate goal is to be a parent, right? This will allow you to fulfill that goal." It was that last sentence that had me unpack the reason I wanted to have a child. Of course, I very much wanted to have a hand at making my husband a father. He also waited all his adult life to be in a situation where he would be in a marriage. He repeatedly told me that he was a product of a divorced household. He did not want this for any of his children so they would not have the problems he faced due to the divorce. I knew the importance of a two-parent household on the development of children.

I recalled the conversation my husband and I had early in our relationship. "I'm an older woman. Conceiving will not be as easy." "We can always adopt," he responded. This was one of the reasons I fell in love with him. I, too, considered adoption as a possibility, but when he suggested it made me realize that I could build a life with this man.

It now made perfect sense to be having a conversation about an egg donor. Our willingness to consider having an adoptive child led us to be more open to a child who would have my husband's DNA (but not mine). It would be just as fulfilling or more appealing for our family. I never stop thinking about how things affect me, my family, and others around me. It's a gift and, at times, a detriment. If we made this decision, would others think of me as a fraud and a phony because I was going to carry a baby from someone else's egg?

Sharing the Origin Story

How would my child react to the idea of coming from another woman's egg? How would I tell my child about his or her origin? At what age would I reveal this to my child? Ages five to twelve are too developmentally young. The teenage years may also be quite traumatic because they are developing a sense of identity. Wouldn't it be devastating to inform my child that I was not his or her mother by genes? What would my family think of me for not continuing their genetic legacy?

This kept me up nights before my daughter was born. I wrestled with how to impart this news to my daughter when the time came. Would my child love me as much as her father? What if she wanted to find her egg donor mother at a certain point in her life?

A Test of Faith

Then there was the question of testing faith. Did God intend for me to take this road in life when it was evident that I could not have a child at my age? Even though I had enough questions and doubts to contemplate for a lifetime, we still decided that the egg donor program was the best course of action at this point. We were excited and frightened at the idea of having our own nuclear (pun intended) family. I knew the road would not be easy, but nothing prepared me for the challenging roller coaster ride ahead of us.

Before I started the egg donor process, I had faith in the Almighty. However, I was not pushed to show how strong my faith was until I experienced five years of disappointments. Despite all of the personal challenges I faced, faith kept me going year after year. I knew deep inside that God made this promise to me because I prayed and pleaded with him for an opportunity to be a good mother, to have a chance to do the hardest work I have ever done, knowing it would be the most rewarding of all.

Along the way, my faith weakened from time to time. Key people gave me spiritual encouragement. These special people had stronger faith than I and would remind me of a God who keeps promises. I found continual support and God's voice in an extraordinary nurse at my NYC facility from the donor egg program. After every transfer failure, Nurse Pamela Rasheed encouraged me. She prayed for me and with me, sent me scriptures and faith worship songs. She helped me up when I wanted to break down in the doctor's office as I felt that other forces were trying to keep me from what God had planned for me.

Nurse Pamela was aware of spiritual warfare, so she often reminded me to hold on and pray as fervently as I could. While preparing for the last embryo transfer, I went through the usual practice of having my blood drawn for the same lab work. Nurse Pamela called me in and gave me a CD. She explained that her pastor had given a sermon a week before and, for some reason, veered off from his message and landed on childbearing – about Hannah in the Bible who was barren but prayed fervently for a child and God answered – her son was the prophet Samuel. Pamela went on to say that she spoke with her pastor afterward, and he admitted that he did not plan to expound on that "childbearing" topic during his sermon but it came to him while he was attempting to make a point about having faith as small as a mustard seed.

I took that CD and played it often in my car from the ride to and from work. This CD gave me more fuel to continue to seek support, do more research, and self-advocate. I stayed up reading articles and watching YouTube videos on the success stories of families who had children through the IVF process. This preeminent expert on women's reproductive health appeared to be speaking about me. I could not believe that he was explicitly discussing how a tight cervix may be a potential factor in poor outcomes for women going through IVF.

Things like this happened to me throughout my quest to have a family. I don't think it was just coincidence that I found that video. I wholeheartedly believe that God led me there. The more I sought God, the more he showed up in places and in people I was not expecting. For example, once I started working more closely with one of the "Fathers of IVF," Dr. David Shapiro in Las Vegas, he would order out-of-the-ordinary bloodwork, which my regular facility did not do. Going to different lab locations to get bloodwork also showed me that more people believed in God's goodness than society has us believe these days. I found that even in those locations, I met believers who would pray with me and acknowledge the strength and love of the Lord.

This level of encouragement was so powerful. It kept me grounded, less anxious, and more undaunted. I felt that God saw what I was facing and was showing up to guide me through these clinicians.

An Egg Donor

Initially, I was ignorant about the donor egg process. If our child was remarkably different from us, it would cause people to ask questions that we were not able or willing to answer. Fortunately, we had a doctor and social worker who answered all our questions regarding the donor types and helped collect a personal account of what we would want as a donor match. I think the donor match was the easiest part of the process.

The social worker even asked for a picture of me. The healthcare team spent time reviewing my specifications instead of my husband's because he would be already genetically tied to my daughter. They gave me as much information about the donor egg patient as was available. I was a bit let down that I couldn't see a picture of her but understood that this was the facility's policy. Things became much more real after we were matched and received word that our donor produced nine eggs.

After fertilization, we had five healthy embryos. It was remarkable. The doubts and reservations did not occupy my mind as in the past. I became preoccupied with when we would see, hold, touch, and kiss our babies. Those embryos were our babies. They were so real to me. I already felt connected to these embryos that will be my babies.

When I had my first official pregnancy through egg donor transfer IVF in 2016, I was ecstatic. It was the first time I had been pregnant through this long, physically, mentally, and emotionally draining process. My embryos were transported from the NYC facility to Las Vegas. In all the five years, I did not have a pregnancy outcome until I started working with Dr. David Shapiro, the specialist in Las Vegas. Dr. David Shapiro used extraordinary techniques due to my diagnosis and severe cervical stenosis. He explained that he could only apply the medical knowledge he has acquired throughout the years, but "God had the last word."

Miscarriage

Can you imagine having a doctor who knew that God had a hand in what was to come? My heart and soul were beyond thrilled to know that this doctor understood that God was my fortress and refuge. While the pregnancy ended in a miscarriage, my angel nurse, Pamela, and the doctor had faith that I should continue pursuing my dream of having a child.

As I look back on how things unraveled, I am still so amazed by the fact that Nurse Pamela knew it would happen. At one point, she explained to me that she had a dream (it could have been visions) of me having children. I was so deflated by the miscarriage that I thought she was just trying to lift my spirits. That was not the first and last time this nurse spoke those words to me. She repeated that to me frequently. Her strong convictions gave me further hope, and I began to see the miscarriage as a sign of what was possible. *I was able to get pregnant* from the donor egg was something we celebrated because I had not experienced that once in all the five years of trying.

Deepening Faith

Therefore, I increased my prayer life, focused on my relationship with God, and tried my best to practice more

Christian values and views. My prayer life was more consistent and meaningful. I also found myself giving back more to my community by volunteering for church activities or giving more time and attention to others who needed it. I studied and listened to the Word of God because I truly had not before. I don't know how others survive such a hard time in life without seeking His presence.

Every appointment and follow-up I had, I prayed. I prayed to not knowingly hurt anyone as I advocated for myself and directed my overall treatment. It was not easy, especially as a layperson in an industry that is overseen by highly educated individuals. I was grateful that my donor IVF doctor, Dr. Brooke Rhinehart also welcomed the idea to work with another doctor. She arranged for the remaining embryos to be transported to Dr. David Shapiro so he could also perform the embryo transfer procedure. I came to find out that her interest was pure and true. She was just as invested in seeing us have a child as we were. She gave us the blessing, which was a relief for me.

Second Pregnancy

I know deep within that it was God's will that we have our beautiful daughter. On April 18, 2018, we found out the second transfer with Dr. David Shapiro worked. I can't explain our joy and gratefulness to be pregnant beyond 10 weeks, finally. I cried and prayed, prayed, and cried. My world was not the same once I knew that our precious little girl was on the way. Every day I experienced emotional highs and feelings of blessings, fortune, and favor.

I also worried about the health of my fetus. My thoughts were, "Here I am, an older woman with a history of miscarriages (two before IVF and one with IVF) and questioning the health of the donor egg." The negative thoughts were always in the back of my mind. Whenever I had them, I prayed and reached out to Nurse Pamela and other friends who could pray with me.

Bleeding

Nurse Pamela was still supporting me in my early months of pregnancy and beyond. I recall that I started bleeding very early on in the pregnancy. Right away, I remembered the miscarriage a year earlier. Nurse Pamela instantly said, "Do not allow the devil to take over. This baby is coming." She was obviously correct.

Even the way I met my OB-GYN was a work of God. A pap smear is part of the regular list of exams that must be completed before an IVF procedure. I didn't have a regular OB-GYN but got a referral for a group of doctors affiliated with my first IVF facility.

My doctor was kind and warm. We spoke about my desire to have children, and she also was open about her medical experiences. She informed me that she worked in a hospital in Ghana, supporting women who were expecting. She and I hit it off. I told her when I was pregnant, I would like to work with her. The kind soul she is, she encouraged me to schedule an appointment with her as soon as I knew I was pregnant.

When I came into her office and told her of my pregnancy, she hugged me as if I were an old friend of hers. I felt such encouragement, love, and an overwhelming level of kindness. All my visits with my OB-GYN went exceptionally well. Our daughter was growing and developing just as anticipated. There were no issues at all.

Although fear and uncertainty were plaguing me, I prayed about it and moved on with the process. Pregnancy slowly chipped away at those doubts. My stomach grew, and I grew in love every month. As my daughter was developing in vitro, I was falling deeper and deeper in love. By the time she came to this earth, I was thoroughly and deeply in love with her.

Hospitalization

It was in the 37th week that things took a turn. I went to my regular visit, which I had weekly by now because I was considered high-risk. My doctor took my blood pressure and saw that it was elevated for the first time in my pregnancy. She sent me for further testing that day, and I did not leave the hospital until a day later. The doctors and nurses worked on bringing my blood pressure down before I could go.

Without missing a beat, my doctor did forewarn me that I might need to have the baby earlier, but I did not put much stock in that since they had successfully decreased my blood pressure. I went to work and return at 2:30 PM the next day for a sonogram. By the time I returned, the healthcare providers told me I had fluid loss and had to go directly to the hospital for delivery.

A Coincidental Phone Call?

It may sound unbelievable, but as I sat in that train seat traveling to the hospital, my phone rang. It was Nurse Pamela – why today, why this moment? It's been months since we spoke. I explained what was going on, and she began to pray. She prayed for minutes for my unborn child, for God to see me through this, and for my health. The phone was interrupted under the subway exactly as Nurse Pamela finished her prayer.

My OB-GYN was in the building but seeing other patients when I got there and expected to leave for a dinner party that night. I guess it must have been the fright in my eyes and lack of trust with the attending doctor that resulted in my doctor make some adjustments in her schedule so she could direct the delivery of our daughter. Here I credit God for intervening.

Why My Husband Was Missing

My husband was nowhere near the hospital in the hours up to my delivery. During my pregnancy, our relationship deteriorated. It was stressful for both of us to receive one negative result after another. There were times we could not eat or carry on our activities because we had gotten an alarming report on the outcome of our IVF procedure. We persevered, nevertheless, because we were both committed to having our family. The two of us decided that we wanted to have a family in a home with both mother and father present.

I was aware of all the research about children of divorce. I wanted my children to have the benefit of both parents. Raising children was tough enough without the absence of one of the parents. Lastly, we were Christians and wanted to ensure we were following God's plan. Before our daughter's birth, our relationship problems just got worse after we moved from one state to the next.

My husband lost his job in 2015 and has not worked since. I was carrying the household bills and all the expenses of the IVF treatments. I felt so alone in my own home. I periodically lashed out at him for not planning better as a man.

My cultural norms have dictated that males are the providers. My father had lost his job at one point in my childhood, but I saw him sending resumes and doing whatever he needed to support my mother. My father was never comfortable with my mother being the sole provider. I too was quite uneasy about being the financial head of the family. The sacrifices I made seemed so severe and unbalanced: all the medications, shots, appointments, my father's death in 2016, and the burden of the financial obligations across the board. It was so stressful at times that I used my work to avoid any interactions with my husband. I stayed late hours even when I didn't have to, just to keep my peace and sanity.

Dealing with the Stress

Thankfully, my stress level didn't jeopardize my livelihood or career. I excelled during times of stress at my work. One thing I learned to do early in my career was to compartmentalize my emotions. It's no mystery; learning to be guarded with your feelings came easily for me. None of my colleagues were privy to my situation except two close work friends who went through IVF. Focusing on others' needs was helpful to me during this time. Working in a public service-oriented organization provided a buffer.

My work took the focus away from my personal problems and allowed me to invest myself in children and families who required it fully. It was so fulfilling to secure services and supports for students who were struggling to engage educationally. Some of my colleagues questioned my unwavering dedication to my work; they were not aware of my inner struggles. Some even suggested that I was seeking a promotion.

Promotion was the farthest thing on my mind. My supervisor approached me about a promotion in 2013. I was not interested mainly because I received promotions two consecutive years prior, and I just wanted to stay put for a while to do the best work I could do. I needed stability more than ever. Whenever I got disappointing news about an IVF cycle not working, I buried myself back into my work.

On some occasions when I came across cases where children were in foster care, and parental rights were removed, I wondered why something like this could happen when so many couples were yearning to have a child or two of their own. My husband's words would also replay in my mind. "We can always adopt."

Financial Stress

Another area of great challenge was the financial burden of IVF. Having the typical IVF treatment is astronomical and added to that was the egg donor program. I used up all my three trials of an IVF cycle, for which insurance was able to pay for a high portion. My insurance did not cover the egg donor program's cost because I was over-age, and we did not have those types of funds saved. Consequently, I borrowed against my retirement plan to cover the sixty thousand dollars I needed to cover the initial cost.

The costs continued to increase each step of the way. I needed more money and resources once I discovered that I had to seek an expert in the field of fertility. Dr. David Shapiro, a world-renowned specialist with over 30 years did not practice in New York where I lived. No, my specialist practiced in Las Vegas. Each trip to see him involved airfare, hotel, and food. The expenses mounted.

The cost of the medications I needed to take in 2016 and 2017 was jaw-dropping.

I drew upon every resource that I could find. This led me into a deeper financial hole. The mortgage and living expenses emptied my wallet and bank account; I maxed out my credit cards. I get constant calls from my creditors regularly asking me when I will make payments because I put everything on credit.

What Can Go Wrong?

The fear of something going medically wrong during the pregnancy was also constant. Given that I was a high-risk pregnancy, the regular visits to the doctor's office were reassuring but also anxiety-provoking. Every time I saw the sonogram and heard the heartbeat of my daughter, I was relieved that she was finally going to be in my arms, safe and sound, until the next visit. The day I saw my daughter for the first time in the hospital was when I stopped stressing about her arrival.

I was the person to whom my family and friends came for emotional and financial support. It was not at all easy to find myself needing others. The vulnerability of it also provided a valuable lesson to me that I shall not quickly forget. My family taught me to keep things close to my chest due to embarrassment or shame. This time in my life, I realized that a problem shared is a problem half solved. Talking to family and friends about my hardships proved to be much better for me in the long run than keeping it bottled up.

My husband either stayed downstairs in our home or remained out all night. There were times when he slept practically all day. By the time I was pregnant, we did not sleep in the same bedroom because of my feelings of betrayal. This was not the typical sense of betrayal a woman experiences when their mate steps out on them. I felt that my husband betrayed the relationship by not owning up to his responsibilities and protecting his unborn child and me.

The Value of Therapy

I also had therapy with a Christian counselor. I learned with my therapist, who immensely helped me. She listened to my fears and knew I did not have any money to purchase items for my child. I admired the way she would speak with countless clients and keep all our different issues separate. She provided the care, understanding, and judgment-free environment I needed.

I had already been hard on myself, feeling deflated at times, and thinking I was a failure in life because of the deep financial debt I had on my head. She tried to instill in me that all I needed was my loving arms, nothing else. I tend to be a realist and did not take much stock in what she said. I kept worry to a minimum. I prayed and continued to speak with my therapist, either weekly or bi-weekly.

My husband and I had limited interactions, and negative communication between the two of us made me quite concerned about what type of environment into which our child would come. Throughout my pregnancy, we did not communicate much or interact on any personal level. We only spoke when it was to chastise or insult each other. I was growing tired of feeling like he was taking advantage of me.

Divorce Proceedings

I found out I was pregnant in April of 2018 and filed for divorce in July of the same year. After I decided that the only way forward was to get a divorce, my husband chose not to have anything to do with the pregnancy, not even attending the prenatal appointments. His excuse was that I would embarrass him at the doctor's appointments. I don't know how quickly most folks complete their divorce proceedings, but ours dragged on for months. It wasn't until November that my lawyer had a court date on the calendar.

My attorney was a kind and gentle man, quite different than how my therapist described him. I expected a hard-nosed, aggressive man. Instead, he was supportive, caring, and able to share a male's perspective on my situation. That was meaningful to me. My concern grew that something was wrong due to his frequent medical appointments. I later discovered that he was going through medical procedures due to cancer. Not wanting to violate his privacy by asking him what type, I was as patient and understanding as possible.

Baby Shower

Two weeks before our daughter decided to make her grand appearance, a few of my coworkers (true friends) got together and held a surprise shower for me. The shower took my breath away. I did not anticipate it; the event was spectacularly glorious. It still brings me to tears that those women thought so much of my child and me. Between my friends at work and my coworkers, I received everything that a baby needed. The blessings flowed. This was only the power of God. God saw me in my situation.

Then she (Hagar) called the name of the Lord who spoke to her,

"You are God Who Sees"; for she said, "Have I not even here [in the wilderness]

remained alive after seeing Him [who sees me with understanding and compassion]?"

Therefore, the well was called Beer-lahai-roi (Well of the Living One Who Sees Me); it is

between Kadesh and Bered.

— Genesis 16:13-14 (The Bible, AMP)

Given my background and all of my other personal experiences so far, I thought I was doing pretty well at handling the level of surmounting stress, but that day in November, after my court date, I was holding on to more than I thought. I had a follow-up doctor's appointment directly after the first divorce proceeding. I landed in the hospital that day.

Hospitalization

I asked my older sister to meet me at the hospital because the relationship between my husband and I was nonexistent. I lay in the bed with my sister sitting in a chair beside me. I stared at a piece of paper with the two names I had decided on, realizing the baby was coming at any moment. As the technicians, doctors, fellows, nurses, and RNs walked in and out of my room, updating me about next steps and attaching items to my body, all of the anger, hatred, and resentment I felt towards my husband just dissipated.

I texted my husband to announce our baby was arriving. I told him the baby's name, and he was so pleased because the middle name was his deceased mother's name. I had no clue that the name I selected was his mother's name. I knew which first name I was planning on naming our child but not the middle. The middle name came to me in the hospital.

It felt like something or someone else was in charge of my every emotion and thought the entire time at the hospital. God was present and continued to show His presence in my life and send me loud and clear messages, especially regarding the relationship with my husband.

Becoming Parents

While we were over the moon with our daughter's arrival, all the incidents that occurred the years before she arrived slowly built a large wedge between us. The divorce papers and court dates were still lingering in the background, while new motherhood and lack of sleep took a toll on me. I cried out to God for mercy and grace because I was suffering from postpartum depression at least several weeks after our daughter's life.

The Nativity Scene

It was too much to bear, I thought back then. Then God showed me the way once again. Our church holds a yearly Christmas pageant where children reenact the nativity scene. This year the church called me and asked if we (our daughter, my husband, and I) could participate in the pageant as Jesus, Joseph, and Mary. I did not miss the symbolism and meaning. The depth of the message God gave me became more apparent when one of my dearest childhood friends sent me a scripture (Matthew, Chapters 1-2) of Mary and Joseph's impending separation when our Lord and Savior was conceived. I could not deny the message, and I certainly was not going to defy God blatantly.

Change of Heart

Ultimately, I stopped the divorce proceedings, and we both focused on our daughter. It is not an easy marriage at this point, but we are blessed to have each other in this ever-changing and complex world. My daughter loves her father and enjoys time with him. Her father is wholly devoted to her. For now, I am comforted and satisfied with that in my life. God asked me to consider a greater love than myself, and my daughter was worth it all.

Three months of maternity leave ended, and we had visited all the daycare centers in our community. We reviewed the prices of nannies as well. God made a way for my sister to stay with us a month as we were still figuring out childcare for our little one.

It was such a painfully hard time for me. I was frightened about leaving our daughter alone, even with family and friends. I wondered how other families did this. Plus, how was I going to afford her childcare costs? I had nothing in the bank after I paid my sister for the month she stayed with us.

New Role for Dad

The exceptionally gifted and intelligent lactation expert from La Leche was the one who planted a seed in my husband's head about childcare. She told the story of her father taking care of her as a child. The lactation expert described the loving and close relationship she shared with her father because he was the caregiver when her mother was at work.

I was quite nervous about the idea of having my husband care for an infant all day. Moreover, I wanted to be the stay-at-home parent. Regrettably, left with no other options, and with the reality that my husband did not have a job, we decided that he would take care of our daughter until I got home. He has been taking care of her since she was five months old. In between this time, my mother came and supported us with caring for our daughter. The blessings continue to flow again and again. Our daughter is developing with love around her, and she is a source of love with everyone.

Now that she is here, she has my personality and smarts (her father would beg to differ). She is such a spunky and fun-loving child. Whether she is mine or not is no longer prominent in my thoughts. The interdependency of love and attachment between my daughter and me is everything I hoped for.

I don't think I would have done anything differently. Sure, some of the pain and hurt I endured could have been lessened, but, on second thought, I would not be the transformed person I am today were it not for those experiences. I have matured tremendously in so many ways. Most important to me is the relationship I've built with my Heavenly Father. I am not a Christian who is well-versed with Scripture (I do admire some of my brothers and sisters who are), but I am gradually and consistently trying to listen to God's whispers.

My Faith

My faith has grown by leaps and bounds from where it was in 2016. I've learned to not harbor grievances against others for long periods. Learning to communicate my displeasure and allowing others also to confront me on my wrongs is an exercise that is commonplace for me now.

Given a chance to advise women on fertility, I would tell them not to allow others to doubt the possibility of God's hand in your life. Do not let others steal your dream of parenting and receiving unconditional love from a child. Everyone's financial situation is different. Despite this, don't be deterred by money issues. For women who are much older and are having challenges such as I had, allow yourself to be open to the possibility of donor eggs. You will never regret it. I guarantee it.

For younger women, if you can marry and start a family earlier, do it. I am not one for young people marrying too early. However, having gone through what I have, I would encourage young women to find a serious partner. The earlier that couples decide to have children, the better. Don't assume or take it for granted that you will have children even at younger ages. Put the energy and effort in finding a decent partner now so that you can make critical decisions. The point is that you will have more room and time (God willing) to plan and take measures if infertility becomes an issue.

Be as intentional about your reproduction as you are about your career if a family is your goal. I would encourage women to hold on to friendships that are nurturing, mature, and supportive. Those relationships will play a major part in your growth and make you realize that family is not only about the genes you share. Sometimes family is the people who are beside you through the storm and sunshine.

Likewise, I encourage you to know that love exists in this sometimes-harsh world of ours. People are outstanding by nature and look for instances to reciprocate kindness and love when they can. While looking for my child, I learned that love was all around me in the form of support, well wishes, and genuine happiness others showed.

Lastly, do not be intimidated by professionals in the field. Consider them your partner(s) and be direct about your innermost wants. Ask questions, especially if you do not understand what is going on. Do your research.

Try to be well informed about your care. I've found that doctors appreciate patients who have some knowledge about their health. You will never know as much as your doctor; however, having an idea can go a long way to helping you advocate for yourself.

I will lift up mine eyes unto the hills, from whence cometh my help.

My help cometh from the Lord, which made heaven and earth.

— Psalms 121:1-2

Chapter 12

ANNABELLE THEISEN

Delight yourself also in the Lord, and he will give thee the desires of thine heart.

— Psalms 37:4 The Bible – KJV

Author's note: Annabelle adopted two embryos for her second attempt with a Frozen Embryo Transfer (FET) and gave birth to twin girls. She said that "writing her story brought back so many memories… and I kind of miss the person I was before the girls! Motherhood is the hardest thing I've ever done—emotionally and physically—and I don't think anyone could prepare you for it!" But now she cannot imagine her life without them. Although it's been tough work, she would not trade it for the world. Here is her story.

I Always Knew I'd be a Mom

When I was a child playing with my dolls watching my mother, I always knew I wanted to be a mom. And I know some women don't have that strong feeling, but I did. However, I never thought motherhood would happen to me the way it did, with beautiful twin girls conceived with donor embryos through IVF in my late 40s. I feel truly fortunate in my experience with IVF.

Going it Alone

The hardest part for me was always knowing I wanted to have a baby, getting older, and not being in a relationship. It isn't a sad story, though. I was living in NYC, working in Rockefeller Center, and traveling the world solo. As a successful editor for an outstanding company, I was happy, but I still wanted more. I wanted to feel purpose and to be a mom. I knew that feeling in my heart came from God, and I had faith it would happen. So, I decided to do it on my own.

When I went to see my OB-GYN at Columbia University Medical Center (CUMC) for my initial consultation, I learned that I had been in menopause six years (much to my shock!) I thought my missed periods were due to stress and over-exercise. My OB-GYN told me I had premature ovarian failure. As I took in this news, I was devastated. She referred me to the reproductive endocrinologist (RE) within CUMC.

Donated Embryos

The infertility specialist at CUMC told me about IVF. I learned I could have either a donor egg and donor sperm or a donor embryo. There were my only choices. I became hopeful because this was something I never imagined was possible.

I found out the embryos available for adoption were donated by couples who have already achieved successful IVF treatment and completed their families. This indicated that the embryos are products from a proven/successful batch. The donating couple did not believe in discarding their excess embryos or submitting them for clinical research.

It was almost a year later that I decided to move forward. I needed time to mourn the loss of never having my biological child, and I had first to accept the idea of the donated embryo possibility and procedure.

I never imagined my life in this way. I wondered what my baby would look like—knowing she or he would not look like me—but I knew it didn't matter. In the end, I yearned to be a mother. I wanted to experience pregnancy—to feel a baby growing in me. It was that clear. I never had the option of using my own eggs. I realized that embryo adoption was the only choice for me as a single woman. Adoption is a long, expensive process that's made even harder for a single woman.

Once I made the decision, I wanted to try IVF. For me, IVF was a dream come true – as this was the only choice I had - and something I embraced. I had faith in God and knew I would be a mother.

First Embryo Transfer

My biggest setback was that my first embryo transfer did not work. I was disappointed this embryo did not implant.

"Why did this happen to me?" I questioned every step in the process because I was so sure it was going to work, but in the back of my mind, I thought, "How many women get pregnant the first time?" I gave myself a few months before trying again. And I knew I wanted to do it differently—both in my thinking and in the experience.

Although I knew the statistics presented to me by my doctor and based on the American Society of Reproductive Medicine (ASRM) data, I still wished that it had worked the first time. "Maybe I need to try something different? Should I ask to be implanted with two embryos instead of one? This would increase my chance of becoming pregnant."

When I brought up the subject, my doctor and nurse explained the risks of multiple babies if two embryos were to be transferred—twins or even triplets or quadruples. They said there was a possibility (less than 5% chance) of an embryo splitting in the early implantation stage becoming identical twins. Another risk of multiple babies was early delivery resulting from complications of gestational diabetes, high blood pressure, and pre-eclampsia.

I knew of women who had premature babies. When babies are delivered prematurely, they are faced with neonatal complications as well, especially complications related to lungs being underdeveloped to sustain life.

I decided to proceed with two embryos the second time around despite the risks. I would rather be pregnant with twins than not pregnant at all.

Second Embryo Transfer

Armed with the sense of being practical, having faith in my doctor and nurse, and weighing the probability, I pressed on towards my goal and did not hesitate to try adopting again. The second time I did a trial run and found out I had a polyp on my cervix, which the surgeon removed. I also did progesterone shots instead of pills. I wasn't afraid of the needle's size or giving myself a nightly injection, which I know some women are. Again, for me, it was the end goal—a baby. I persevered.

The second embryo transfer procedure went so smoothly, a much different experience than the first. I felt it was going to work and prayed it would. This time I was more relaxed than the first. I didn't analyze every little twinge. I stayed positive and tried not to get my hopes up, telling myself I would try again if it didn't work. And 10 days after my transfer, I received a call with the results of my blood test.

The Phone Call That Changed My Life

"Congratulations, you are soooo pregnant!" I couldn't breathe. I couldn't believe I was pregnant. I didn't feel any different. My HCG levels were good and high, and stayed that way. A few weeks later, I found out I was pregnant with twins – both embryos took. I then learned that they were girls. I thought about how they would have each other as best friends. I was so happy. I never imagined my life in this way. And knowing the girls would have each other was very special.

I knew that having twins was a possibility based on what the doctor said, the success rate she discussed, and what I had read before and during the process. But I didn't know what to expect—especially after my first cycle with one donated embryo didn't work. Based on the data, will transferring two embryos this second round fail, lead to singleton, twins, or triplets?

The team at Columbia University Medical Center was amazing. My doctor and the nurse assigned to my care made me believe that this was possible for me. And of course, my faith made me strong, and I believed that I would be a mother.

What was also noteworthy was that my nurse, Pamela (the author of this book), was also a woman of faith, and she encouraged me even during the difficult periods of the process. However, I didn't tell my family members and friends right away. How do you explain your attempt at pregnancy with donated embryos when you are trying to come to terms with it? What if it fails? However, when I did disclose my pregnancy and how it was made possible with donated embryos, they supported me.

My Fears

My biggest fear was about the survival of the girls. At first, I kept praying the girls would grow, and I wouldn't have a miscarriage. When I knew the girls were healthy and developing as expected, I was relieved and excited about being pregnant and knowing I would soon be a mom. I was a little worried about what a c-section would be like and how I would feel afterward.

My Success

Thirty-seven weeks and six days after that phone call, I gave birth to two beautiful, healthy girls. I was finally a mother. My life is not the same – I feel fulfilled.

My biggest challenge was when the girls were newborns. Taking care of two small newborns alone was hard, especially as a sleep-deprived new single mom. Also, I never expected the feelings of loneliness and isolation. Motherhood is such an emotional journey; you give birth to a baby and to a new self. And to compound that, you are single and far away from close relatives – this phase was difficult.

Speaking as a successful single woman who became a mom in my forties, I can say that I always knew I wanted to be a mom. I just didn't know how it would happen, and never imagined it would be in this way. The only advice I would give is to be open to the possibility and ways in which motherhood can happen and have faith that it can.

To him that will, ways are not wanting.

— **George Herbert - 1820s**

CHAPTER 13

PRUDENCE AND NATE SMITH

There's always a light at the end of a tunnel but the way out is through.
— DAVID ALLEN

When I got married at the age of 33, I was happy and hopeful I would be blessed with all the joys of marriage. My faith led me to see myself as a mother. However, my situation was difficult because my spouse lived in a different country, and it would take some time before he could legally migrate to the USA.

Reunited

After three years from the time we got married, and by God's blessings, my husband relocated to the USA. We were excited to be together finally and to start our family. We expected that we would conceive rather quickly, but unfortunately, that did not happen. We sought help from a doctor, who said that we needed to try on our own for one year, and if we didn't conceive, then I could return, and the team would do further investigation.

A year passed without success, so we went back to the doctor. After numerous tests, I was diagnosed with fibroids;

my doctor advised me to have surgery, given the fibroids' positions and sizes. The doctor counseled me that the fibroids would make it exceedingly difficult for me to get pregnant and give birth.

Seeking Financial Help

My team referred me to another hospital for the surgery. Luckily enough, I had a successful fibroid removal. I went back to my doctor, and he suggested that I start fertility treatment, but we did not have the money needed because we were low-income earners. I discussed our financial dilemma with my doctor, and he got me enrolled in government programs in New York for low-income earners who had difficulty conceiving. It took about a year before we got approval for the grant.

No Success

During this year, I had no success conceiving on my own. We needed to undergo more tests to make sure I was a good candidate and strong enough to through all the processes. After the successful testing process, my doctor started treating me with Clomid, since that does not cost a lot of money. I was on the medication and under monitoring by blood tests and ultrasounds for three cycles to determine the ovulation's appropriate time. We tried but failed yet again.

My doctor then suggested artificial insemination for another three cycles, which did not work either, so my doctor said we should go for IVF. My biological clock kept ticking. I started to become more disappointed and scared and questioned what the problem with me was.

Eventually, we gathered our resources and took a loan, at which time I finally started the IVF treatment. I felt so lucky; we got nine eggs, some fertilized, and we ended with two "strong and active embryos," according to the doctors.

Success

The transfer took place, and two weeks later, we heard the wonderful news: "You are pregnant—finally!" God has been so good, and I thank him. My husband and I were so happy.

I gave birth to our beautiful and healthy baby girl.

Second Attempt

We hoped to have more babies. My doctor then advised me again not to wait too long to try again. After I stopped breastfeeding my baby six months later, we went back to the hospital to start the necessary paperwork as before and pay for another cycle. Because of my age, I didn't get enough eggs like the previous cycle. The team retrieved six eggs and fertilized them, but that yielded only two embryos. They weren't like the last cycle. Instead of day five for transfer, the doctors said we must wait one more day and do a day six transfer. The very day I was going in for the transfer, while on my way, I got a call with sad news. "The embryos did not survive. Go back home." I was devastated. I started to cry. How could this happen to me? I was despondent and broken.

What Are Our Choices?

After we put all the pieces together and gathered our shattered emotions, we went back to the hospital to plan again. My doctor said that because of my age, there was a possibility that my eggs would not be as healthy as when I was in my teens, so he suggested that we should try donor eggs. The financial cost was too much for us to consider this option, and we were still paying off the previous IVF loan.

The doctor gave us another option, which was the donor embryos. It was difficult for me to decide, but I thank God for my husband, who did not think twice. Eventually, we agreed to accept an embryo donated by another person to help us have another baby.

We went to the hospital and met the doctors and the co-ordinator in charge of donor embryos. After completing all the necessary paperwork, we reviewed our preferences, and paid the money, much less than we expected. The embryo was a gift, but we needed to pay for the monitoring ultrasounds, blood tests, and doctor's fees. I began the treatment, which was like the previous ones except for an egg retrieval. I started the injections as usual until everything became ok for the transfer. It was successful.

"You Are Pregnant" and I Am Miserable

Two weeks after the transfer, I went back to the hospital for a pregnancy test, and once again, I was pregnant. Now I was supposed to be the happiest woman on earth, but I was not. I became extremely paranoid, thinking maybe the doctors made a mistake and transferred an embryo different from my preference.

I was anxious, depressed, and felt guilty, wishing I was not pregnant. Questioning my spiritual values, I thought I had committed a sin against God, and now I was being punished. Sometimes I asked myself, "What if the baby came out to be Chinese, Asian, or a different race? What would people say? My church would think I committed adultery." Also, I kept asking myself, "What if the baby grew up and found out that I was not his/her biological mother?"

So many questions tormented me. I could not eat or sleep as I became more paranoid and depressed. Because of these thoughts, I called the hospital and explained everything to the coordinator in charge. She suggested I should see a therapist. She quickly made an appointment for me. I saw the therapist yet did not feel better.

I called the coordinator and told her I wanted to abort the pregnancy. She then asked a nurse to speak with me. That is when I met Nurse Pamela, who listened attentively and gave me words of encouragement. As she was of the Christian faith, she continuously encouraged me with words from the Bible, and she prayed with me. She has continued to stay in touch with me.

My husband was overly concerned about my wellbeing and became worried for us. He encouraged me to exercise some patience. He told me everything would be fine with time; he was a great source of support. It got to the point that his words became my source of hope. After five months, my anxiety and depression calmed down, and at the seventh month, I gave birth to another beautiful and healthy baby girl, who added to the source of my happiness.

We cannot imagine our life without her. My older daughter has a sibling; they have each other, and they love each other so much. My baby girl completed our family. Our home is filled with love and joy, and we are forever grateful for this gift of God.

> *Trust in the Lord with all your heart*
> *and lean not on your own understanding;*
> *in all your ways acknowledge Him,*
> *and He shall direct your paths.*
>
> **— PROVERBS 3:5-6 (NKJV)**

Chapter 14

Rochelle and Damian Henderson

Science and technology have come a long way in overcoming barriers to natural conception, and we give the credit to man's intelligence, but ultimately, it is God who gives life.

— Pamela Rasheed, MSN RN

Author's note: Speaking as a nurse at the heart of the third-party program of the infertility clinic where most of these beautiful stories occurred, this is a story of Divine Providence. Every story shared by these families is very dear to me because I believe I was placed in the paths of these women for a purpose. I genuinely believe God set me up for this one.

This story reveals how a woman's desires, coupled with faith, met with science and triggered a series of events that could have only been orchestrated by none other but God to make this woman a mother.

A Fateful Meeting That Changed My Life

I was in my early fifties when I met a woman in my community by chance or perhaps by God's providence. My husband and I tried for several years when we were much younger to have children but with no success. In an era when insurance did not cover assisted reproductive technology such as IVF, we spent all our savings. We had insurmountable credit card debts trying to have just one baby. After three years and the loss of much money, time, and hope. After an unsuccessful attempt at IVF, we lost the battle.

We were emotionally and financially depleted and could no longer pursue becoming parents. Yet I wanted to be a mother and wished I had a child of my own. As a teacher who spent so much time around children, the pain of not having a child of my own, coupled with the everyday reminder of my failure, overtook me. As a woman of faith, I thought that I might be a mother one day, but now I realized it was no longer possible.

The Overhead Conversation

In the summer of 2016, I attended an event in my community and overheard a conversation among some women of the local church. These women were complimenting their Bible teacher on a lesson she taught from the Book of Ruth. The lesson they discussed was called "Was Ruth Barren?" In that conversation, I overheard the teacher said that she was also an infertility nurse, which made her master that topic. My ears perked up – the nurse's comments stirred up my lingering desire for a child.

At the end of the conversation, I approached the Bible teacher, who worked at a well-known university hospital in New York. "Do I understand that you work as an infertility nurse?" After the conversation where I detailed my prior attempts at IVF, she offered information about adopting an embryo.

This was startling and intriguing. I had never heard of becoming pregnant and delivering a baby to call my own from an embryo donated by someone else. This was mind-blowing. I asked, "How could this be? Was this fate?" I prayed and realized that my desire to be a mom had not perished with my aging, depleted funds, and loss of the will to try again. Maybe these events were orchestrated by God.

I was a newcomer at the same church the infertility nurse attended. In hindsight, I realized the pastor's sermons during that season were words he spoke into my life. As I talked with others, I learned this Bible teacher who showed kindness was not just "an infertility nurse" but rather "THE Infertility Nurse" who headed the egg and embryo donation program at this prestigious medical center.

This was a kaleidoscope of events that led to this perfect situation, the ideal timing of a God-orchestrated faith incident – this must be divine providence.

After learning that I could not have a child with my own eggs and my husband's sperm, but that I could adopt an embryo, become pregnant, and carry to term, I began to feel hope. The nurse shared success stories of her prior patients and cautioned me that I must be healthy enough to do all the above, and even so, there was still no guarantee. I decided to take my chances because my wishes to have a child were still alive.

My husband, who already had a child from a prior relationship, was incredibly supportive. I got his full support, and now I was determined to do whatever it would take. The procedures would not be so costly as other IVF treatments I had gone through with my own eggs. Although I was sure this was God's way to grant my desire, I had to apply that faith and continue my journey.

The Journey Begins

The initial consultation with the infertility doctor took place just two weeks later. A series of blood tests, ultrasound, and evaluations by maternal-fetal medicine specialists began. Ultrasound revealed that multiple fibroids in my uterus and a myomectomy (surgery to remove fibroids from the uterus) was necessary.

It was not an easy journey. First, there was a uterine factor, and I needed surgery to remove fibroids, a setback I did not anticipate. Fear set in, and I began to question, "Is this worth it?" I felt uncertain and wondered if I was now on a wild goose chase. Should I accept my fate as is and stop pursuing this dream? Nevertheless, I was on the path, and nothing was going to stop me now.

I waited in the patients' lounge to talk to my nurse after learning about the need for surgery because I needed a voice of reasoning. Nurse Pamela assured me that surgery, regardless of how scary it might sound, was just a routine procedure for the experts involved in my care. It would enormously benefit me. With encouragement and clinical guidance, I plunged deeper into the journey of having a baby at any cost.

The surgery was successful, and the matching process for an embryo began. The "wish list" that I needed to complete detailed the characteristics and attributes that I desired and required in my baby, such as ethnicity, etc. I learned the embryo I would be matched with was a "gift" given by a couple who had completed their family with the desired number of children, but who did not want to destroy the remaining embryos.

After the embryo match, we needed to pay for the procedures to assure we would receive an embryo.

Embryo Transfer

Within one year from the day I initially spoke with the nurse, I was scheduled for my embryo transfer. My clinicians always reminded me that although the embryo was from a successful batch, there was no guarantee that it would result in a positive pregnancy. Even if the pregnancy test was positive, there was no guarantee that the pregnancy would result in a live birth.

Was I doing the right thing? Should I stop? Should I save myself the heartbreak of failure and further loss of money? "No", I reasoned. All the series of events that had played out over these past months were signs that this was my season. God would stay true to His promise – my faith took over and led the way.

"You are Pregnant"

Two weeks after the embryo transfer, the blood test revealed I was pregnant. I was elated. I expressed my gratefulness and said, "Indeed God is faithful and true to His word!" I repeated the pregnancy hormone test (beta HCG) every two days and heard the good news each time from my nurse that beta-HCG levels were rising appropriately. I became more confident that this was indeed my season, my gift, the fulfillment of God's promise to me.

Bleeding

However, as I waited to attend my first pregnancy ultrasound, I began to bleed. I panicked and needed reassurance I would be OK. I called Pamela early that Sunday morning. Though hopeful, Pam had to manage my expectations appropriately and honestly by telling me this bleeding episode could either be an unfortunate miscarriage or nothing concerning.

Pamela explained that the reason for bleeding in early pregnancy is often not understood and may not lead to a miscarriage but that it was hard to tell without further evaluation. The ultrasound that day confirmed my baby was OK: my baby was inside the uterus, there was a heartbeat, and the measurements corresponded to the dates.

The doctor and Pamela decided that if a positive fetal heartbeat and all the initial markers of a healthy pregnancy were evident at the second pregnancy ultrasound, Pamela would tell me she had accepted a new position with a different company. This was Pamela's last day (of ten years) in her job at this infertility clinic.

I sat up on the examining table, not knowing what to say. Pamela said, "This was it, Rochelle. I was here for this very event, and now it's fulfilled, and I am released to a newer season." Without a shadow of a doubt, this was orchestrated for me – from that first meeting in the community to this day. I was walking in a season of motherly bliss, one I could have only imagined until the God I trusted in showed up and fulfilled my deepest longing.

I delivered my healthy baby boy in 2019, and my life has forever changed to right side up, in my fifties. This is truly a story of faith, science, and God's gift. Often, I ponder this and ask, "Who would have known and who could have brought this to pass for me but God?"

For I know the thoughts that I think toward you, says the Lord, thoughts of peace and not of evil, to give you a future and a hope.

— **JEREMIAH 29:11 NKJV**

For with God, nothing shall be impossible.

— **LUKE 1:37 KJV**

Chapter 15

Nola and Brian Anderson

*It is understood that the beauty of a rainbow
does not negate the ravages of any storm.
When a rainbow appears, it does not mean that the storm
never happened or that we are still dealing with its aftermath.
It means that something beautiful and full of light
has appeared in the midst of the darkness and clouds.
Storm clouds still hover, but the rainbow provides
a counterbalance of color, energy, and hope.*

— WWW.SMALLBIRDSTUDIOS.COM

When it is not getting pregnant as the issue but keeping the pregnancy — just keep swimming.

From an early age, I always had a desire to be a mother. As a child, I would spend hours "mothering" my baby dolls: dressing them, feeding them, and brushing their hair. I just knew that one day I would be a mother. What I didn't know and couldn't even begin to fathom as a young girl, was that I would encounter heartache, heartbreak, and character-building life lessons.

Meeting My Husband

When I met my husband in 2009, I knew he was "the one." He is smart, patient, loving, and quite family-oriented. Moreover, I knew he would be a good— scratch that—a GREAT father! After years of dating (and one long period away from each other), we finally got married in the winter of 2016. Almost immediately, I became more intentional about growing our family, taking prenatal vitamins, tracking my cycle, eating right, and working out. Ten months into our marriage, I asked my husband if he was ready to start officially trying. He said he was, and so our journey began.

First Pregnancy

As fate would have it, one month after that talk, I found myself pregnant for the first time at 36 years old. I was BEYOND excited. I was finally going to be a mother. I had read stories of women around my age who had to try for months or years before becoming pregnant, and I thought, "Whew! I dodged that bullet." I could hardly believe it. When three home pregnancy tests came back positive, I quickly called my OB-GYN to make an appointment and started making plans for our future child; I was so excited.

No Heartbeat

At my first OB-GYN appointment (around six weeks), we reviewed my medical history, and I had my first ultrasound. AND THERE IT WAS, our baby's heartbeat. It was surreal. With the pregnancy confirmed, I was walking on Cloud 9. I told my husband, and he was very excited, as this was going to be his first child. Three weeks later, we returned for our ninth week check-up, and that to this day remains one of the worst days of my life. Our little baby... our little joy... was no more. There was no heartbeat.

How could this be? I had seen the heartbeat a few weeks earlier, and it had looked strong. I was devastated, hurt, and confused. Between big globs of tears, my husband and I made the appointment for the dilatation and curettage (D&C) to remove the dead fetus. The date was March 2, 2017. After my D&C and subsequent healing period, I became even more obsessed about growing our family. At my post-D&C follow-up appointment, my doctor assured me that "these things happen" and were fairly common, and to not give up hope of becoming a mother.

That turned out to be easier said than done. With every passing month and negative pregnancy test that followed, I felt a piece of my heart and soul crumbling away. I wanted THAT baby. I loved THAT baby. I was mourning for THAT baby. And truthfully, to this day, I still mourn for THAT baby.

Acupuncture for Fertility

Fast forward to the summer of 2017. While I wasn't completely worried at this point in my journey, I became more concerned and, again, intentional in my pursuit of motherhood. So, I decided to give acupuncture a try because I heard that it could boost fertility. I researched and found a practice 10 minutes from my house that specializes in acupuncture for fertility. I called, and as luck (or fate) would have it, they were accepting new patients. I made an appointment for a consultation.

I feel that now is an appropriate time to let you know that I am a woman of faith. I believe in God, and I know that I am a friend of God and that Jesus Christ is my Lord and Savior. There have been many times on this journey (and in my life in general) I felt God's mighty and powerful hand stitching the pieces of my life together. He has been and continues to be my sustainer, my rock, and my shield. And I genuinely believe that every step on my journey to motherhood was specially orchestrated and ordained by God. He indeed turned my test into a testimony. And for that, I am forever grateful.

I genuinely believe the day I walked into that acupuncture practice, my journey to motherhood shifted. Now don't get me wrong, I was still in for many more months of heartache, of wishing and praying for a baby. But on that day, there was a shift. My acupuncturist was truly heaven-sent. She did more than just stick me with needles. She listened to my fears, wiped my tears, gave me wise counsel, and encouraged me to keep going.

IUI

In early 2018, after one year of trying to conceive, my husband and I began fertility treatments at one of the best reproductive clinics in New York. By June of that year, we had undergone three unsuccessful IUIs, resulting in one complete failure and two chemical pregnancies. By this time, I was completely beside myself. I was starting to believe that all was lost. Maybe I wasn't meant to be a mother after all. But I knew that wasn't true. I knew this hope and burning desire to become a mother was a promise that God placed in my heart.

My Diagnoses

At this point, my acupuncturist recommended we see a maternal-fetal medicine doctor. This highly regarded and respected doctor had developed a reputation for helping women like myself who were able to conceive but, for some reason, were not able to maintain the pregnancy. After a battery of tests, my husband and I finally had an answer as to why we had suffered several losses. I had a form of thrombophilia (increased creation of factors that lead to clotting) and elevated natural killer cells.

Both conditions worked together to attack (like cancer) any pregnancy I could conceive as explained to me. The doctor recommended I begin his natural vitamins and supplements protocol to stabilize and prepare my body for a successful pregnancy.

Second Pregnancy

I started the protocol at the beginning of August of 2018, and after many months of negative tests, I conceived again naturally. I felt like we had finally received a second chance. And to my surprise and delight, at our first ultrasound, we learned that the egg had split, so I was carrying identical twins.

I remember being happy but very nervous and anxious. It was as if I knew something wasn't quite right. Well, I was right. I miscarried both twins a few weeks later, and my second D&C took place on October 24, 2018.

The next three months were probably the lowest points of my journey and our life altogether. The ache in my soul for my lost babies (all five of them—yes, I count the chemical pregnancies) was too much to bear. I was angry, felt hopeless, and could not understand why this was happening to my husband and me. We were good people. Why was the Lord punishing us? I leaned on my faith like never before.

Positive Pregnancy Test

This journey brought me closer to God, and it humbled me in a way that I never knew possible. I questioned everything, up to and including Him. So, I continued with the vitamin and supplement protocol, and in February 2019, we conceived naturally again on our third anniversary. I took a home pregnancy test on March 2, 2019, two years to the day of my 1st D&C. It was positive.

We'd been here before. But, this time, there was a strange peace and calmness that overcame me. This pregnancy felt different. After bloodwork and ultrasounds confirmed the pregnancy, we approached this pregnancy with cautious optimism. Could it be? Was this one going to stick? I remember, for weeks, going to the bathroom and praying with every wipe, "Stick, stay, grow!"

On October 24, 2019, one year to the day of our 2nd D&C for our twins, our rainbow baby, a healthy, strong, and beautiful baby boy, was born. He is, for us, God's promise incarnate. He is my constant reminder that God hears our silent prayers, never wastes a hurt, and keeps His promises.

Are you a woman reading this and wondering when it will be my turn? When will I get off this roller coaster called (in)fertility? I say, "Never give up hope. Always believe in the power you possess just one more time. Be gentle with yourself. Be kind to yourself. Love yourself. Talk to someone. This burden can get so heavy at times. Talking to someone can help to lighten that weight."

And if you are a believer, pray and trust Him and His will. The struggle with (in)fertility is a monster that can steal your joy and mess with your mind and soul in the worst ways. I'm here to remind you that you are whole. You are NOT broken. You are not alone. You have an entire community of warrior women rooting and cheering you.

Remember, the journey and path to motherhood can take many forms—none are cookie cutter or perfect—but all are designed to reveal our inner strength and resilience. And on your worst days, remember what Dory in *Finding Nemo* always said, "Just keep swimming" because tough times don't last always, but tough people do!

For the LORD God is a sun and shield: the LORD will give grace and glory: no good thing will he withhold from them that walk uprightly. O LORD of hosts, blessed is the man that trusteth in thee.

— Psalm 84:11-12

Chapter 16

Dustin and Caren Moore

Author's note: In my conversation with Dustin Moore I learned that he and his wife experienced the heartbreaks from recurrent pregnancy losses, including three sets of twins. They have done several rounds of IVF and FET, got pregnant each time but miscarried each time. Dustin and his wife adopted a baby girl early in 2020. As an enormously proud father, he shares his story.

*To humans belong the plans of the heart,
but from the Lord comes the proper answer of the tongue.*
— **Proverbs 16:1 NIV**

"A couple flying home with their newly adopted daughter received an impromptu baby shower on the plane," said an article published in the CBS and other news media on February 13th, 2020.

I reached out to new dad Dustin after reading his story. Dustin and his wife have gone through so much to have a baby, but when all else failed, and their desire continued, they turned to adoption. He boldly declares that it is not that his daughter, who is the blessed one to have been adopted, but they are the ones blessed to have her as their daughter.

New dad Dustin Moore admitted on Twitter it had been a tough week. The California nutritionist didn't want to air his grievances on social media; he wanted to turn the mood around. So, instead of talking about his hard week, he shared a story about a recent day, the day he and his wife brought their new daughter home. "I hope our story uplifts you and reminds you there is goodness to be had in this world," Dustin Moore wrote on Twitter, diving into the heartwarming tale.

"Not too long ago, my wife and I boarded a Southwest Air flight with our recently adopted infant daughter," he wrote. When the couple boarded the plane, Moore apologized to his fellow passengers, as many parents with babies feel pressured to do while flying. "About mid-flight, our daughter awoke and politely informed us she wanted a new diaper," Moore's Twitter thread continued.

"After inquiring about space for a table change, a thoughtful flight attendant (named Jenny) cleared a space in the back of the plane and gave us privacy." The flight attendant also gave the Moores a set of pilot wings for their baby girl, who, as an infant, had already experienced flying. Then, the Moores learned that the two kind flight attendants, Jenny and Bobby, were a couple, too. "We learned they were married, and that someone had done a similar act for them on their honeymoon flight," Moore said. Jenny wanted to pay it forward, just like the act of kindness they received on their honeymoon.

"Even as we disembarked, people kept approaching us and wishing us well, and complementing our beautiful daughter," Moore wrote. "Our hearts were full."

"But there's more. What all those perfect strangers and attendants did not know was the emotionally tender state of two brand-new parents," he wrote. "Parents who, after nine years of trying, had been blessed with their first child, parents who felt scared but determined in their new role. The outpouring of love from that flight brought on by the actions of two thoughtfully observant flight attendants... it exceeds my ability to describe what it meant to us," Moore continued. "How much those wings and written notes uplifted two new parents determined to love their new daughter."

Dustin shared an image of a photo album where he and his wife have stored all the notes they received from strangers on that flight. "(Twitter) is often used as a means to share what's wrong," Moore wrote. "I hope you'll take time to share what is good."

Moore said he and his wife were at first concerned about how people would feel about them and their adopted daughter. "We were insecure about people not thinking much of our daughter," he told CBS News. "It's not very rational, but we were just concerned about what people would think by virtue of her being adopted by us. We didn't give birth to her. But the fact that that entire flight, everybody cheered, everybody took the time to share those notes with our daughter, it was just everything we needed at that moment just to feel secure and to feel, 'Okay, this is going to be great,'" he said.

A man's heart plans his ways, but God directs his steps.
— **Proverbs 16:9 KJV**

Trust your creator and take Him with you on your life's journey.
— **Pamela Rasheed, MSN, RN**

Part Three

THE HIDDEN COSTS

Chapter 17

Relationships and Truths

Couples often are united at the initial consultation with the infertility specialist, but most end up on a lonely journey and sometimes alone over time. Being alone is quite different than being lonely. Cohesiveness in infertility is related not only to a sexual relationship but also to all other human relationships. People can be in a relationship that appears to have all the appropriate boxes checked but still feel alone. Even though it seemed that my coupled patients were together, they were quite lonely in their misery of infertility and felt alone in both marriage and outside their marriage. These are a few areas that take a hard hit, resulting in relationships: support, self-blame, and guilt.

Support

Some couples may be supportive of each other. I have observed this mostly when both female and male factors contribute to the inability to conceive. However, a partner's support dwindles significantly when the failure to conceive rests upon the other's infertility diagnosis alone.

If couples accept that the infertility diagnosis, whether male or female etiology, is a unified diagnosis, they may be more supportive. One factor that causes one to feel less supported is the notion that "unless you are standing in my shoes, you won't know how I feel," while the other might say "I am not the one with the problem" often sending a psychological and emotional blow to the other.

Parents, siblings, relatives, friends, employers, and even clinicians and religious affiliates affect the couple's perception of support. Couples faced with infertility tend to keep it private and often withdraw from others and events that may remind them of their difficulty conceiving naturally and easily. Often, their withdrawal is because of feeling judged and unsupported by both the people they care about and those who provide care to them.

I have encountered judgmental members of both clinical and religious teams. A coworker thought that because a patient had a couple of abortions before her current relationship, she was punished through having difficulty conceiving.

I heard a religious leader say a woman with infertility was being punished with recurrent losses because she aborted a fetus. (She chose to end a pregnancy that involved a fetus with a severe genetic disorder.) As you can imagine, women especially may feel less supported, isolated, and alone in their fertility journey, not only from their partners but also from others.

The lack of support is not one of those issues that is typically addressed during infertility treatment. Women or their partners need to seek other therapies such as support groups and psycho-therapy. Lack of support leads to feeling sad, and a woman and/or partner may become depressed if they do not address the root of these issues.

Tips from the Infertility Nurse

Acknowledge and thank the people who make you feel supported. If you feel unsupported in your relationship, try to talk about it with your partner or someone you trust. Avoid being around people or sharing your infertility struggles with those who don't understand because their honest effort to make you feel better can make you feel worse. Some of the things they can say that would inadvertently make you feel less supported and sadder are:

- "You can always do IVF."
- "You can just adopt."
- "Trust me; you're lucky you don't have kids."
- "Maybe you're not meant to be a mom or dad."
- "What's the big deal?"
- "This is not the end of the world."

These people may just be trying to make you feel better when these comments are upsetting. It's best to get support through expert counsel and empathetic support.

Self-Blame

Blame is a big game that gets played fiercely behind closed doors by both males and females, depending on who has the primary diagnosis of infertility. Keep in mind that one in every ten Americans of reproductive age faces an infertility diagnosis, and men make up approximately a third of the infertile population, according to the American Society for Reproductive Medicine (ASRM).

The person with infertility issues often hears, "It's your fault!" This blame is displayed, not only in words alone but also in a partner's body language and overall behaviors. In my years in the clinical setting, I have often counseled the patients to try empathy in understanding that men and women view infertility differently.

Studies and clinical observations concluded women experience more significant infertility-related stress, are more likely to blame themselves initially, and face depression and anxiety. Also, women take treatment plans more seriously and are more likely to be more disappointed when treatment fails. The male partner should try to understand the different perspectives of the grief process to be more supportive.

A man deals with infertility quite differently than a woman. Chapter 2 refers to country singer Chuck Wicks and his wife Kasi's struggles to have a child. "Chuck was crushed to learn the issue lay with his sperm. 'As a man,' he says, 'the issue is: the last thing you want someone to tell you is you can't do this. It makes you feel small. It makes you feel like you're not a man.'" He became depressed, and his wife had to encourage him while they pursued a medical solution (Kruh, 2020).

In her story (Chapter 11), Sadie said she slept in a separate bed and only interacted with her husband to berate him. This display of emotions is often a result of blame, coupled with a lack of support. Unfortunately, it is quite common in the world of infertility, but the healthcare providers often do not address it. Blame rips into the fragment of a marriage like a wildfire and often cause irreparable breakdowns of trust and wholeness. Though a successful outcome of infertility treatment may occur, the pain and scars linger.

Tips from the Infertility Nurse

Remember your marriage pledge, "For better or for worse." Put your "Couple Power" to work and avoid faulting your partner; you are a "one-unit" structure now. Get an outside perspective by seeking counseling from a professional, psychologist, or faith-based person if needed, but don't let self-blame or the impulse to blame your partner dominate. If either of you had the choice, you would not choose your diagnosis – it's there to be dealt with and overcome, not to engulf and overtake you.

Anger

Anger causes couples to inflict deep emotional and psychological wounds on each other and can ultimately lead to a breakdown in their relationship, hence a more stressful journey and ultimate failure. Blame leads to anger, and anger leads to an inability to cope with the diagnosis and seek treatment effectively. Experts concur that unless anger is identified and reduced, it festers. Angry feelings not only lead to a break down in relations but also create an unreceptivity to pregnancy. As documented in the chapter (Chapter 24) related to alternative medicine, it is essential to have all parts of the patient in synch: mind, body, and spirit.

Tips from the Infertility Nurse

First, acknowledge that your feelings of anger, grief, anxiety, and uncertainty are real. Be honest about your feeling with your partner and be open to hear his/her part even if silence is all you hear. Speak with someone you trust. Talking is an outlet and does not keep your thoughts and emotions pent up. Talking is healthy (even when talking to the person in the mirror) as it lets you hear yourself as your own voice of reasoning. It is even alright to shed tears. Crying, whether privately or on the shoulders of a friend, serves as an outlet and is a healthy coping mechanism. This method allows you to understand your options.

Join an infertility support group. Your clinic may offer support groups, and Resolve.org is a popular one.

Chapter 18

The Reality of Stigma, Grief, Shame, Fear, and Uncertainty

It is an understatement that assisted reproductive therapies are easy. The biological technology is groundbreaking, and adequate clinical resources are ever-present. Infertility treatment is not as focused on support for the emotions such as grief of not conceiving naturally, fear of being childless, and uncertainty about treatment outcome.

Additionally, there is a sense of loss in dignity and pride. Barrenness is still a reality that is shrouded in shame and guilt, and it impacts the expectations a person has about being a parent. The wife of Chuck Wicks said she had three daughters from a previous marriage, and when she married Chuck, she could not imagine *not* having a child with him" (Kruh, 2020).

How can partners with an infertility diagnosis combat these issues in addition to potential stress on their marriage or relationship (where applicable), and allow their mental and emotional biases to tap into the tranquility they need to function in the infertility world? In cases of a woman's male partner's infertility diagnosis being present, she may also feel these stressors.

First, a layer of shame needs to be peeled away and exchanged with the initial acceptance of the diagnosis that renders them infertile as a couple. The couple who has the resolve to move forward has won half the battle. I often speak with women who experience grief over their loss of having a baby the natural way. After they overcome that, they move on to treatment. They face the disappointment of a failed treatment cycle. Eventually, the initial stage of grief and disappointment subsides with either a positive outcome or a resolve to keep trying.

Further failures lead to rips in the fragment of self-esteem. A couple experiences negativity and threats to their marital relationship, further breaking down their emotional and psychological resolves. A couple needs crucial support on all levels possible – from family and friends, bosses and co-workers (if they are willing to open up to them), from workshops provided by the clinic, and from organizations such as Resolve.com. Sadie (Chapter 11) told me about the support she received from her co-workers – they threw a surprised baby shower for her and the utmost support brought her to tears.

The process of undergoing the many steps of infertility treatment is draining. Comedian Michelle Buteau found nothing funny about enduring five years of IVF and four miscarriages. She said, "We were at the end of our road in terms of me trying." After she found a surrogacy agency, her dream of becoming a mom came true. Michelle and her husband Gijs van der Most welcomed twins carried by two surrogates. "These women are like walking angels on earth," she says, "I text mine all the time. Just like, 'Thank you'" (Strohm, 2020).

Consider the stigma and shame of the following woman. She struggled privately and did not seek treatment became of the stigma and shame of being labeled "barren." As a woman of faith, she counts herself blessed to have conceived after eight years. She said:

> "Having children, whether pre-planned or accidentally, is derived from relationships. More so, traditional family units carry this expectation. While the Western culture may force couples to wait before having a child, a traditional culture consisting of a patriarchal setting will pressure couples to pursue childbearing. As such, the norm of starting a family and having children is a given despite their financial status, educational privileges, or physiological maturity. Therefore, childbearing is paramount. The female is the main one responsible for bringing this cultural truth and expectation to fruition.
>
> The underlying issues within that culture will surface when a couple married for a standard period cannot conceive. Because of fear of what others might think, the couple may keep personal matters private even when infertility gets to a chronic stage. Moreover, when a couple cannot conceive, people often do not approach with a listening ear or clinical remedies. They are more quickly to

presume that something may be drastically wrong with the female.

As a result, many couples and particularly women, become isolated from others and much-needed help. Over time, the shame of infertility can cripple any marriage and relationship.

Females are at a higher disadvantage of being labeled barren more than men. The stigma that follows a couple can pressure their health and well-being, catapulting the couple into a spiral of seclusion, depression, loneliness, bitterness, and self-hatred. Eventually, infertility is not the only factor they are battling, but other factors, when added together, can put any relationship into a spiral of chaos, confusion, and destruction."

Tips From an Infertility Nurse

It benefits the woman to open up to someone who will not be judgmental but will listen and acknowledge her concerns. A place to begin may be with your primary doctor – a GYN or a PCP. The next step will become easier eventually; a visit to the infertility specialist will be a bit more bearable. At this time, consider sharing with someone you trust to keep your secret and to be supportive. Every step taken becomes more comfortable, and eventually, you would have covered much distance than you thought.

Although the other layers of finances, socioeconomic, social, psychological, and spiritual dimensions get added, and the burden becomes heavier, keep the goal of having a baby in sight. This is easier said than done and consider the need to seek non-clinical interventions such as counseling or alternative therapies and medicine (Chapter 26).

The Roots of Stigma and Shame

Stigma and shame are rooted in a person's culture and often cause isolation and demoralize patients. The patients are left to battle these feelings alone, even when they are in healthy relationships. Over six million women in the U.S. of childbearing age battle infertility and most of them feel the stigma while enduring the sting of shame. Many push through the shame and guilt to achieve pregnancy regardless of the obstacles; they suffer stigma in silence.

Culture is the embodiment of beliefs, lifestyle practices, values, and traditional groups' expectations. People's cultures affect the choices they make about infertility treatment. Therefore, clinical specialists, nurses, and other support staff need to understand and consider their patients' cultural differences within the clinical settings.

Aarti and Neil

Consider Aarti and Neil's situation and how they coped with their unexpected diagnosis of premature ovarian failure (POF). Aarti was a thirty-six-year-old banker who was married for three years when she learned of her POF diagnosis. She was shocked. In her culture, women do not openly talk about their sexuality and marital relationship challenges, so talking about difficulty conceiving is shameful. As a result of POF, Aarti internalized her grief and remorse when her healthcare providers told her that an egg donor would be her best option for becoming a mother.

Instead of pursuing this route, Aarti allowed herself to get lost in her job and excelled professionally. Her marriage fell apart, and now in her early forties, she is bitter. Her relatives feel the sting and some of Aarti's friends drifted away. Aarti was reluctant to continue infertility with donor eggs because she felt that her relatives would eventually find out and label her as barren, in addition to possibly berate her for having a child who's not genetically her own. She did not want to seek therapy and was reluctant to attend workshops related to her diagnosis. She got a dog instead and moved across the country.

Neil said, "To be diagnosed with infertility is like being unexpectedly hit with a curveball." No one ever saw this coming. The couple's friends and families waited for Aarti to become pregnant. Their culture compounded their grief over the failed opportunity to be parents. Without the benefit of counseling or family support, their marriage failed, and they did not proceed with having a baby together.

Aarti was too ashamed to reveal her diagnosis to her family and friends. Others would frown upon her for the need to use an egg donor to have a baby. Additionally, if her husband divorced her and got other women pregnant, her family would realize she was barren. Combining these factors resulted in her suffering the shame and stigma associated with the inability to have children without an egg donor. This is not easy to fix unless she can get over the cultural pressure and expectations.

General Expectations

Common beliefs and practices are deeply woven into the cultures of people. These factors affect ideas about fertility and the role of a couple to produce children: demographical, religious, racial, sexual, egotistical, and social. These beliefs and practices define people and impact their life's choices, including having children. When looked at globally, culturally, and socio-economically, the differences in perception and access to infertility care affect childbearing.

As a result, those who face an infertility diagnosis *may* pursue some types of infertility treatment. For example, a devout Catholic might not undergo IVF due to a religious belief. Some highly religious people believe life begins at fertilization. Excess embryos from an IVF cycle may be discarded, which is against that religious conviction. The disposal of embryos was a hot topic and a point of opinion and debate during Justice Amy Coney Barrett's Supreme Court nomination hearings 2020.

As another example of controversy, a man may not be willing to submit to clinical evaluation in the diagnostic phase because that is an exposure and threat to his manhood. He may have a potential male infertility factor, but because of the cultural belief and practices ingrained in him, an infertility diagnosis will make him "less than a man."

A culture may assume the woman is "always to blame" for a couple's inability to conceive, thereby setting up a roadblock in her male partner's clinical evaluation. Unfortunately, even when the woman alone is evaluated and found to have an issue, not knowing if there is also a male factor will result in failed treatment and a negative impact on the couple and their families.

Social Implications

Society may see men and women as inadequate or inept if they are not able to conceive naturally. In many cases, they may not want to discuss their diagnosis or struggles with friends and family. Sometimes they shy away from events that remind them or call attention to this inadequacy in their existence, such as at family gatherings and children's birthday parties.

Infertility causes a decline in self-esteem and gradually tears away the social well-being of a person. Some societies may look at a woman as "less than" if she did not fulfill her most natural biological expectation of childbearing. This aspect of infertility is a sensitive one, and when family and friends are not aware of the condition of a loved one, they may make remarks or gestures that can cause pain. It is also essential the clinical staff is sensitive when treating the infertile person or couple.

Traditional Expectations

In Aarti and Neil's case, they are both Indian immigrants with large families. Their culture dictates that they, too, must have children. This culture does not openly discuss sexuality or marital struggles as its members keep personal matters private. When these two factors are combined, Aarti and Neil developed a sense of failure and needed to keep the reason for not conceiving private. Their private struggles and lack of support may have caused their marital breakup.

Tips From an Infertility Nurse

Understanding and overcoming the *stigma barriers* related to infertility involves first identifying the origin of these factors. Consider whether they are rooted in your social, cultural, or societal areas of life. This may help you pinpoint a more productive way to deal with them. Once you find out the root of these feelings of inadequacy and reluctance to seek support from family and friends, you can then acknowledge how these factors make you feel in dealing with the diagnosis of infertility. Address the root cause and move on to seeking the support – it is available.

Reach out for support by speaking with a counselor. Absorb the techniques an expert may recommend and empower yourself to overcome the stigma and shame. Do not let these non-biological factors add extra layers and negatively impact the physical setback because it is the biological realm (diagnosis) that requires your primary focus.

The broader community can be a source of help in reducing stigma. When notable people or celebrities openly discussed their fertility journey, it helps to destigmatize this element. When former first lady Michelle Obama openly talked about needing IVF to achieve pregnancy, it sparked a rise in women of color to seek fertility treatment.

Like Sarah Jessica Parker and Kim Kardashian, many celebrities openly spoke about surrogacy, sparking a greater interest in this option. Some states revised their laws as necessary due to women who need another woman's uterus to carry their babies. When notable women become vocal about these issues, legislators and insurance companies act on the information.

Chapter 19

Financial Implications

Financial aspects can profoundly affect the quest for children. Jacqueline and Rosa had something in common. Each was an older woman who had diminished ovarian reserve and a newer and younger husband. The women felt they needed to save their marriages by making their husbands fathers.

Meet Jacqueline, a forty-nine-year-old clinical psychologist, mother of two daughters in their early twenties, and wife of a new and much younger husband. Jake wants to have his own kids.

On the other hand, Rosa is forty-seven years old, mother of three grown kids, and two grandchildren. She is the wife of a much younger husband, who is twelve years her junior. Now he also wants his own children.

Both Jacqueline and Rosa embraced their diagnoses and the need to be fair to their new husbands who do not have children of their own. Although Jacqueline's and Rosa's situations are remarkably similar, they are in significantly different financial brackets related to affording the cost of a donor egg IVF treatment cycle.

Jacqueline can afford twenty-seven thousand plus dollars for an anonymous or partially known donor IVF cycle with pre-implantation genetic screening (PGS can be gender selective). Jacqueline and her husband prefer to have a male child, whether the cycle fails or not.

Rosa does not have that economic privilege. Rosa's adult daughter will be her egg donor, saving about approximately eighteen thousand dollars in donor fees, medications, and PGS fees from the cost of her egg donor cycle. Cost is a major factor for many such as Rosa, but to what extent is one willing to go? She sacrificed the moral aspect (using her daughter's eggs) in her quest to carry a baby for her younger husband.

What is common in these two scenarios is the need to use donor eggs. Both have children from their previous relationships and come from a culture more open to their need to provide offspring for their husbands.

Financial stress provides a significant barrier in the infertility field due to insufficient insurance coverage. According to most insurances' criteria, having a baby is not a matter of life and death but somewhat optional. Planning is essential but quite different from other achievements, such as buying a house or planning college tuitions. With time, fertility declines, and the probability of success also declines with age.

Tips From an Infertility Nurse

Some infertility centers deemed "Center of Excellence" by health insurance organizations often received government financial grants to assist low-income families paying for IVF. Women who qualify for grants (normal egg reserve is a criteria) are encouraged to ask the financial counselors for any information about this potential financial assistance. Other organizations such as WIN-Fertility also offer a direct-to-consumer (DTC) discounted bundle rate that can be competitive. There are other options, such as borrowing from retirement investments and home equality lines of credit. These options must be taken with risks as there are no guarantees that any treatment cycle will be successful.

Chapter 20

Spiritual Impact: God, Faith, and Religion

Jesus looked at them and said, "With man, this is impossible, but with God all things are possible."
— **Matthew 19:26**

I am a specialty nurse but also one of faith. I believe in the power of science and technology and the Holy Bible, as it presents many accounts of miracles that have served to let us humans know that there is a God with whom nothing is impossible. To those who trust him, there is no disappointment. The principles and stories in The Holy Bible guide me in my nursing duties. As I venture out to work, I want to fulfill my responsibility, not only as a nurse but also as a nurse who believes in miracles.

I believe that God can turn a bad situation around for good like he did when he turned water into wine at the Canaan's wedding (John 2:1-11). This happened for Sadie (see Chapter 11) as she mentioned it in her personal story. In Chapter 14, Rochelle experienced the Providence of God. Her story was a well-orchestrated plan by unseen hands to grant her the miracle of her son when she was over 50 years old.

The year that Sadie became a candidate for egg donation, I became the head nurse of the egg and embryo donation program at a prestigious university medical center in New York City. In her forties and diagnosed with Sjorgren syndrome and diminished ovarian reserve (DOR), she experienced the heartbreak of several failed attempts of IVF with her eggs. Her fertility doctor told her the only option of having a baby would be with donor eggs. Her husband wanted a child as much as she did. However, Sadie, needing to face her diagnosis's reality, grieved in ways that put a wedge in her marital relationship. Nothing he said or did for her was enough to diminish her pain of being barren and her sense of failure as she continued to drift into a place of despair and aloneness. Her husband grieved in his own way.

Sadie became angrier and consistently lashed out at her husband for everything. As the nurse at the center of her care plan, I picked up on those cues and could tap into the depth of her grief – and it was not pleasant. But God had his eyes on them, and little did she know, her Creator saw her, and His ear was attuned to her desperation.

Her husband faithfully came to most of the appointments but did not say anything. I surmised that he remained quiet for fear of being degraded by his wife for sharing an opinion when he was not the one with an infertility diagnosis. Over several years of trying to conceive, their relationship became so unbearable that they filed for a divorce during her pregnancy with her daughter.

To backtrack, they accepted the journey of egg donation, and out of five embryos, they failed two frozen embryo transfers (FET). Sadie became pregnant on the third FET. I remember giving her the good news and continuing to monitor the beta HCG (pregnancy hormone) levels every other day. But before she got to the pregnancy ultrasound appointment, she started to bleed. I planned for her to come in for an emergency ultrasound, educating her that sometimes bleeding in early pregnancy does not ultimately mean miscarriage. Bleeding in early pregnancy is common, and the reasons are not fully known.

Unfortunately, the ultrasound revealed that Sadie had a miscarriage. "Oh, how much can I take?" she cried. The doctor offered her condolences and potential next steps. I did not know what to say. As the nurse who knew more of what Sadie was going through, I offered my support, and I stayed to hear her vent and cry. I listened to her anguish even though she couldn't express it in words. Her eyes were glazed with pain and uncertainty. She said again, "I don't know how much more I can take."

Sadie was out of money; her marriage was falling apart. She was walking a thin line at work, and her relationship with her mother and sister was strained. After hearing her out, I gave her the clinical instruction for further monitoring and advised her to take some time to grieve. At this time, Sadie said that she did not know if she would do this again – she was also emotionally exhausted. Several months passed. Sadie's other two embryos were cryopreserved, waiting on her decision.

One Sunday, Sadie was strongly on my mind for no apparent reason. The sermon that day described how Jesus turned water into wine and the role that his mother, Mary, played when she begged Jesus, saying, "Please help, we ran out of wine." I saw myself as Mary saying to Jesus, "Sadie is out of energy (wine) – please help."

Suddenly, the preacher swung from "Water turned to Wine" to Hannah, a barren woman in the Old Testament of the Bible whom God promised a child, Samuel. I felt compelled to get a copy of this sermon on tape to give to Sadie, convinced that there was something spiritual behind this day – for Sadie, a patient I have not seen or heard from for several months. I planned to call Sadie the next day and asked her to come by my office to pick up this tape, not knowing how she would respond. Would she feel that I invaded her privacy?

- Would she reprimand me?
- Would she threaten to report me to my supervisor?
- Was I risking crossing the line between my professional boundary into her private territory?

I took the risk.

God compelled me to contact Sadie. I took a deep breath, called, and invited her to the office. To my relief, she promised to be there. Little did I know that her marriage was irrevocably broken, and the day she came by my office was her court date with her estranged husband. I shared a summary of the sermon as she began to cry. She said, "Oh,

Nurse Pam, if you only knew what I am going through," as she showed me the envelope of court documents. I did not know what to say, except, "Can I pray with you?" I felt compelled to go beyond my "nurse" duty.

Sadie was in a dark place but still reachable by the Hand of God. I prayed. Sadie cried throughout the prayer. She left my office there knowing that something had changed for her. I felt at peace and knew that God would see her through this – He has her in the palm of his hands.

Sadie's next FET gave her beautiful daughter created especially for her – they are meant for each other forever.

> *Where can I go from Your Spirit?*
> *Or where can I flee from Your presence?*
> *If I ascend into heaven, You are there.*
> *If I make my bed in hell, behold, You are there.*
> *If I take the wings of the morning,*
> *and dwell in the uttermost parts of the sea,*
> *even there Your hand shall lead me,*
> *and Your right hand shall hold me.*
>
> **— PSALMS 139:7-10**

Chapter 21

Psychological, Moral, and Ethical Impacts

Patients face hard choices when donated gametes, donated embryos, and adoption are the only possible roads to conception and parenthood. There are imminent psychological, moral, and ethical implications. These factors become evident from the inception of the treatment plans.

Donor Eggs

Many women who are perfectly capable of carrying a pregnancy to term hit a roadblock if they do not have a good reserve or quality of eggs. Other factors are diminished ovarian reserve (DOR), premature ovarian failure (POF), endometriosis, advanced reproductive age (ARA), and recurrent pregnancy loss.

Rosa, her husband, Juan, and Rosa's daughter (Diane) from her previous marriage, came to the clinic to propose this plan. Diane, Rosa's 24-year old daughter, would be her egg donor. This process is "Known Donor Egg IVF". Diane would go through the stimulation with daily injectable medications for IVF. She would have her eggs harvested to be fertilized with Rosa's husband's sperm (Diane's stepfather's sperm) in the lab to make embryos for Rosa. Here is the family tree:

- Juan would be the father of the baby.
- Diane would be the biological mother of Rosa's child.
- Rosa would be the DNA grandmother of the child she would carry to term, also making her the birth mother.
- Diane would be the big sister of a baby who came from her egg.

Rosa and Juan welcomed a healthy girl after providing legal consent and psychological clearances. They are thinking of a sibling for baby Ava by using a frozen embryo from Diane's batch.

On the other hand, Jacqueline and Carlos are both in the healthcare profession and understand that because of her age, Jacqueline cannot easily have a child of her own. The risk that Jacqueline faced was losing her much younger husband to a fertile and younger woman. (See Chapter 19.)

As a result of her divorce from her first husband, Jacqueline acquired a substantial settlement. In the process of recovering, she met Carlos, fifteen years her junior, at the gym where they both worked out. Carlos was an EMT (emergency medical technician) by night and nursing student by day. He has not fathered a child and did not think it would be a problem.

But several years later, when most of his friends and peers with children started to make comments to him about having his own kids, Carlos began to think about it. Jacqueline had the money – lots of it – and dreaded losing Carlos.

The team at the clinic gave Carlos and Jacqueline an overview of the anonymous egg donor program. Carlos knew he would be a doting dad, but Jacqueline was unsure what concerns she felt and how her grown children's reaction would complicate her fears and perceptions. One year later, they were parents to their baby.

Excess Embryos

Patients who undergo IVF and complete the number of children they desire, or for other reasons, are sometimes left with remaining embryos. Clinics send them a yearly bill of about $1200 for storage of those embryos. Each time they get a bill, they must weigh their options regarding what to do about the excess embryos.

- Should they keep paying storage fees?
- Should they discard the embryos?
- Should they donate to science research?
- Or should they donate to another couple?

This dilemma is not an easy situation, and the decision can be emotionally and psychologically complicated.

A blogger and author, Jamie Sumner (2020), wrote an emotional "good-bye" letter to her remaining embryos. She said in this letter, "It's not how we imagined our lives, or yours, after fighting so hard to get you." She donated her embryos to other couples but promised in her letter, "I will always look for you on the playground and the school hallways on Parent Night."

What should a couple do with embryos once they achieve their goal of having a baby? Some couples believe that once fertilized, the embryo has the potential for life. According to their beliefs, the couple should not destroy these potential lives. Therefore, couples donate their remaining embryos. Most couples would rather give these embryos as a gift to others struggling with infertility who cannot afford egg donation IVF. (Without a donated embryo, they would not have a chance at parenthood.) Additionally, parents who donate embryos achieved their desired number of children. They genuinely seek to allow their embryos to have a chance at life while blessing another woman or couple with the opportunity to become parents too.

When Jo-Ann's nurse asked her what she wanted to do with her remaining embryos, she stated that she was "very torn." Jo-Ann read stories of clinics that are grappling with the issues of abandoned embryos. However, Jo-Ann didn't think that she would ever face a situation of choosing to discard or donate her remaining embryos because it did not occur to her that she would have embryos remaining from her donor egg IVF.

After much thought, Jo-Ann replied, "I want to put a smile on the face of another woman, the same smile I have on my face now." She donated her embryos. She did not want to abandon or destroy her children's potential siblings. Jo-Ann had the number of children she desired, both a son and a daughter. Because Jo-Ann was an older mother with financial strains, she and her husband could not pursue another pregnancy. She recalled when signing the consent forms before her donor egg IVF treatment, she and her husband knew they could discard the remaining embryos, donate them to research, or give them to others. Their gift made happy parents of other couples.

In a society such as the U.S. where assisted reproductive technology (ART) is at an all-time high, many women are prepared for family building at an advanced age (older than 35). Some insurance plans offer infertility treatment coverage such as frozen embryo transfer (FET); it is reasonable to pursue a donor embryo plan. Traditional adoption of children is priceless but often more tedious. Potential parents can widen their options with embryo adoption as well.

According to an article in the NY Times (Hecker, 2020), American IVF clinics are grappling with an increase of abandoned embryos and loss of fees. Moral, psychological, financial, and spiritual choices force couples to decide to donate or discard embryos. Whose embryos are they? It can be complex. Some embryos may be a combination of:

- A woman's own eggs and her partner's sperm,

- her own eggs and donor sperm,
- her partner's sperm and donor eggs, and
- donor eggs with donor sperm.

Tips From an Infertility Nurse

Embryo donation/adoption is a widely known choice. FDA regulations govern biological tissue transplant/transfers. Although most older women do IVF, fewer of them are likely to have excess embryos. A greater number of available embryos would likely come from egg donor cycles where the eggs source is younger. Some of these couples donate their remaining embryos for research while others discard them. It is worth exploring this option with your infertility clinic.

If your fertility clinic does not have an embryo donation program, you can contact the Snowflakes Program. It may be difficult, but the first step in contacting this organization is a great start. Snowflakes has been helping with embryos adoption since 1997. This was shrouded in secrecy, but not so much now as notable people are vocal about being barren and needing help. This program empowers couples to choose life for their excess remaining embryos, giving hope to those who would otherwise not be able to fulfill their desire to have children.

Sperm Donation

Sperm donation has been available much longer than egg donation, and like egg donation, most sperm donors are anonymous. However, some donors are known to their recipients directly or as just an acquaintance. A sperm donor may be a brother-in-law, a friend (gay or straight), and sometimes, a prior sexual partner.

For example, Rocker David Crosby donated sperm to singer Melissa Etheridge and her lesbian lover, Julie Cypher. The couple birthed a son and daughter. Crosby commented, "It was very kind of them both to let me spend time with the kids because our official deal was that I signed papers relinquishing parental rights of any sort after I made my gift. They're great kids; they're very special people in my life." After Etheridge and Cypher broke up, Etheridge married actress Tammy Michaels, who gave birth to twins using an anonymous sperm donor (Wenn, 2006).

In a known sperm donor arrangement, a psychological evaluation and legal contract become part of the preliminary workup. In the State of New York, if a legal agreement is not in place, a known sperm donor can be responsible for child support until the child is 21 years old.

Sperm donation may seem to be a much simpler transaction than egg and embryo donation. Still, there is also a more significant psychological impact on male-female couples where the male partner has infertility. He also experiences loss, grief, inadequacy, and failure of manhood. The treatment plan should include a psychological evaluation to determine how the male partner might react to raising "someone else's child."

Poonam and Gopal entered into a "love" marriage against the Indian tradition of their parents hand-picking who each should marry. (The practice of "arranged" marriages still happens in India.) After two years of marriage, Gopal's firm transferred him to its headquarter in New Jersey. Eventually, Poonam joined him, and as soon as they settled in New Jersey, they began planning a family.

After a year of failed attempts, they consulted the fertility doctor and discovered that Gopal had no sperm in his ejaculate. A urology consult established that Gopal had non-obstructive azoospermia (low or no sperm production that was not caused by a blockage of some sort).

Poonam had an excellent egg reserve – her AMH was 3.44 ng/nl at age 32, and her Fallopian tubes were open. The first line of treatment was intrauterine insemination (IUI) with donor sperm. The second treatment line was a more invasive IVF treatment utilizing a testicular sperm extraction (TESE) procedure that surgically extracts sperms cells to fertilize Poonam's eggs. The cost can range from $3,000-$12,000. IVF with intracytoplasmic sperm injection (ICSI) would be needed, bringing the overall cost of one IVF cycle above $18,000. There is no guarantee of success as the TESE may fail to yield enough normal and acceptable quality sperm. After much discussion, they proceeded with IUI using donor sperm, and Poonam conceived with the first attempt.

Four years later, they returned to have another IUI cycle with the additional vial of donor sperm that remained cryopreserved at the clinic so they could have a sibling for their son. Observing the love-bond and chemistry between Gopal and his son was amazing – little Akshay was more a daddy's boy than one can imagine. He is loved and spoiled by both sets of grandparents who visit the USA annually to be a part of his growing up. Poonam and Gopal, believing their parents would not understand and accept the process by which they became parents, chose not to reveal the secret.

The use of donor sperm has become quite commonplace. In some cultures, it is less stigmatized because of the rights and privileges of the LGBTQ community. IVF and artificial insemination might use donor sperm. Since the passing of laws supporting gay couples' rights to have children, same-sex female couples seek an infertility specialist claiming that they unsuccessfully attempted to achieve pregnancy with at-home-insemination from a known donor. Some insurance plans require a "duration of infertility" (DOI) or exposure to sperm before allowing a patient to access to her infertility benefits. These plans might not recognize undocumented at-home-insemination as proof that the patient tried and failed to conceive before asking for the infertility benefits. Many insurance plans require a set number of inseminations in the absence of a proper infertility diagnosis to move on to more invasive and costly treatments such as IVF.

Janet could not fathom how she ended up at this place in her life – single with a ticking biological clock. When she found out she had a diminished ovarian reserve, she was shocked. Janet became pregnant naturally at age 33 but terminated the pregnancy because the baby's father was not ready to have a child. She did not anticipate the termination would leave her feeling empty, fearful, and defeated.

As a Catholic, Janet thought that she was being punished for that abortion. Grant, her boyfriend at the time, did not seem to care. She recalled his nonchalant statement, "I am so glad we didn't continue the pregnancy." That comment broke her spirit. She hoped Grant felt the void she felt but that not the case. She suddenly realized that she was the only one feeling the emptiness. Janet and Grant broke up.

Although Janet's health insurance would cover the procedure to thaw and fertilize her eggs that she froze several years ago, she would have to purchase donor sperm. With a decline in her fertility rate, simple artificial insemination might not be as successful. Janet embarked on her journey to do whatever it took to have a shot at becoming a mother. Her nurse encouraged her to "have fun" going through the sperm donor profiles at the sperm bank – she got to choose many attributes of her anonymous donor. She could select tall, dark, and handsome with blue eyes, etc.

Janet has always been a high achiever both academically and professionally, but she felt like failure at 40 years old, single and childless. Of the 11 eggs she cryopreserved at a younger age, 9 were fertilized with donor sperm. Of the remaining 7, only 2 were normal. She had her FET cycle in 2019 and delivered her son. In her own words, "I did what I needed to do, and it does not matter that I had to use a sperm donor."

Chapter 22

Anonymity, Current DNA, and Genealogy Testing

With the growing industry of current DNA, genealogy, and genetic identity tests, it becomes less simple to hide family secrets. [DNA stands for deoxyribonucleic acid. It is an acid in the chromosomes found in the center (nucleus) of the cells of living things. It contains the genetic codes of that living creature, and it is unchangeable.]

The path to parenthood through donor gametes, donor embryos, and adoption is a dream come true for many infertile couples. But keeping the DNA origin shrouded in layers of secrecy is threatened by the many available DNA cheek swab, saliva, or blood tests. Today's most significant concerns in the light of DNA technologies are the shattering of anonymity and exposure of secrets that have driven infertility medicine for decades.

A simple saliva or blood test can identify a person's DNA origin. Children born from donor eggs, donor sperm, or donor embryos can quickly discover that their parents are not their right biological link. This discovery can be shocking to the child, and trust may be forever broken.

In her memoir entitled *Inheritance,* Dani Shapiro (2019) shared the emotional and psychological consequences of discovering through a genetic test the man she thought was her father was not. Her mother used donor sperm to conceive her. There are many more stories like this of shock and betrayal. Parents need to find a way to disclose this information to their children at an early age and in a sensitive manner.

Readily available genetic testing is obtainable from sites like 23&me.com and Anescestry.com. The secrets they reveal demonstrate why it is essential to discuss the DNA origins of children. The genetic reports allow matching and finding blood relatives or determining paternity results. In infertility treatments, the secrecy surrounding the use of donor eggs, sperm, and embryos leaves too much at stake when families do not disclose this vital DNA information of their children.

Confronting the Bonds

Prospective parents should consider these questions:

- Will I love this baby even though the gametes, embryos, and baby are not DNA-related to me?
- Will the baby have genetic traits that are troubling or affect future generations?
- Will the baby resemble me, and if not, how will that affect how people react to the baby and me?
- How will the children respond later when they find out about their origin?

In my patients' experience, most of their trepidations are reduced by utmost love and purest joy once their babies arrive. The greatest struggle becomes if and how to disclose the DNA origin to their children.

A family adopted their son Jack when he was a year old. At age 24, he was diagnosed with leukemia and needed a bone marrow donation. In the chaos surrounding this urgent need to find a match, they had to disclose the truth of his DNA origin. Not only did the disease and prognosis weighed heavily on the family, but the truth was shattering for their son and the extended family. Accusations of betrayal required the family to undergo in-depth counseling and healing. The last time I spoke with Jack's mom about two years ago, she discussed how devastating the revelation was for her son. Jack was very intent on finding his biological parents as he tried to grapple with his genetic discovery. His mother felt the threat of losing him. They had to work through the remorse and find forgiveness, which quelled the shocking discovery. Jack is doing better each day..

Tips From an Infertility Nurse

When your children are old enough to understand, use a practical and honest approach to discuss their DNA origin. Let them know of your desire to have them and the medical challenges you faced that led to your choices. Acknowledge their questions at the time and throughout their lives if they need to know more. They must know how much you long ed for them. They were conceived with the generosity and goodwill of another person who had a loving heart. Assure them that they have filled your life with love and life's greatest fulfillment, and you could not love them anymore if they were genetically related.

Perhaps decades ago, it was a best practice not to tell children born of donor gametes how they were conceived, but research shows honesty is the best policy. Children who are told earlier in life will not think it a big deal and will embrace honesty above all else. But children who find out much later are not only shocked by the truth but feel betrayed and angry, especially if they find out by chance, a life's event, or by DNA testing.

Parents must consider that life's secrets are a burden that can be quite heavy; secrets do come out somehow, no matter how long that takes. Family surprises often undermines trust and stability within the family unit and will affect future generations. Parents should relieve themselves of that heavy burden and enjoy their life and relationship with their kids. Kris and Emily Burns, the parents of an embryo frozen for 20 years, said as their son grows up, they would be transparent about how he was brought into the world. "It's never going to be a secret," says Emily (Sechtin, 2020.)

Refer to books about how to tell children they were adopted. You'll find the language you can apply to your own situation.

Also, when famous people and celebrities become parents via IVF using a donor egg, sperm or embryos take the initiative to be transparent about their journey, most of their followers may not feel the sting of the stigma that comes with infertility. When this famous population of women and couples talk publicly, their followers listen, embrace, and imitate.

Chapter 23

Fertility Preservation: The Non-Infertile Population

Fertility preservation is a procedure remarkably like IVF but not specifically for the "infertile" population. A woman not yet focused on family building can save her eggs while she is young rather than wait to find out when she is of advanced reproductive age (greater than 35-years-old) that she has an infertility diagnosis such as diminished ovarian reserve (DOR).

It does not make medical sense for a 40-year-old woman to freeze her eggs because both her egg quantity and quality will decrease to almost zero. In such a case, it is appropriate to freeze embryos – even if donor sperm is the only sperm source option. The healthcare providers will genetically screen the embryos to rule out chromosomal abnormality – rather than freezing eggs alone as a form of fertility preservation.

The WHO's definition of infertility prompts physicians to discuss fertility options such as egg freezing treatments. When a younger population take advantage of freezing eggs, it is an "elective" preservation. Although most insurance plan cover "medical" eggs freezing (in cases of cancer treatment which threatens fertility), only a few insurance plans cover "elective" egg freezing while others do not.

In recent years, infertility facilities hosted "egg-freezing" parties to attract and educate women about their fertility and its rapid decline after age 35. Egg cryopreservation (freezing) cycles do not need sperm because the eggs are frozen until the woman is ready to commit to a male partner. As a result, younger single women do most egg-freezing cycles.

There is no such rush for men to freeze sperm because of aging out.

Many women and men need to freeze their eggs or sperm because of a cancer diagnosis and impending chemotherapy and radiation treatment. This is "medical" preservation, and because this is medically necessary, most health plans will cover the cost. Additionally, a few organizations, such as the Livestrong Foundation will also assist with medication coverage. Like elective egg freezing cycles, this population may be young single males and females. Eventually, they may try to conceive naturally if there is no "infertility diagnosis" and use the cryopreserved eggs only if there is a low egg reserve or another related diagnosis.

When there is a cancer diagnosis, patients may opt to freeze embryos instead of eggs and sperm, respectively, as the success rate of live births from frozen embryos is much higher than the pregnancy rates from frozen gametes. The famous quote in the infertility world is "fresh is better."

This is because eggs and sperm are not optimal when they must be thawed, survive the thaw, fertilized, and implant.

An egg cryopreservation cycle is like an IVF cycle, in that the female must be screened, go through injection, surgical egg retrieval, and recovery phase like in IVF.

I admire and compliment my female patients who are proactive in taking charge of their fertility. This population of younger accomplished women is smart in being strategic to take advantage of this option to preserve their eggs when they are more ready to have children. They show themselves to be responsible by keeping the end in mind from the beginning and ensuring they have achieved their education, career, and life partner before conceiving. The current trend is such that women are much older by the time they achieve these life goals. Therefore, they are more likely to face difficulty conceiving if their ovarian reserve is low or develop other infertility-related diagnoses.

Tips From an Infertility Nurse

Women approaching their mid-thirties who are not yet partnered and desire to have children will benefit from this option. Do not be ashamed or afraid to ask if your insurance plan covers elective egg freezing. If your health plan does not provide this benefit, find out from your gynecologist or a reproductive endocrinologist about out-of-pocket costs.

Chapter 24

Alternative Medicine and Its Impact on Pregnancy Outcomes

Infertility is a complex diagnosis; age is not the only or main factor. This journey can be a lonely one even for couples because they, although coupled, feel alone. As a result, the even more extraordinary complexity of both male and female's emotional and psychological health takes on a new definition. In addition to dealing with advanced age, egg, and sperm factors, emotional stress dominates. It is like the stress experienced by patients with cancer, heart disease, and so on, because it brings an inevitable sense of loss, grief, and uncertainty. Stress inhibits any treatment process. Hence, there are complementary alternative treatments available such as acupuncture, massages, herbs, and Chinese Medicine.

A holistic approach to infertility management involves more than pharmaceuticals and pure clinical care and interventions. Per data from a meta-analysis on "Chinese Herbal Medicine for Female Infertility," Ried and Alfred (2013) stated that "Alternative medicines such as Traditional Chinese Medicine (TCM) might address some of the needs of women experiencing infertility that are not met in the Western medical approach."

As an infertility nurse in the Western world, I often consider that the West is more pharmaceutically driven. How much better would the infertile population be if the healthcare system paid closer attention to the alternative approach and added this complementary aspect into the patient care plan? As a recipient of regular acupuncture, massage therapy, and herbal supplements for my overall wellbeing, I take the initiative to recommend them to my patients, friends, and coworkers for the mere purpose of self-care and reducing stress. A holistic approach has proven to be more effective in synching all the moving parts into a healthy balance.

There are numerous clinical and spa facilities in the U.S. that cater to the infertility clients. For example, in New York City, The Holistic Medical Center and Yin Ova Center, to name a couple, offer traditional Eastern therapies for almost everything that ails the body, mind, and spirit. Infertility is a diagnosis that affects all these areas of a person. As a nurse working in this field, I understand it well enough and would like to incorporate it into our care for this population. Infertility clinics may see their pregnancy success rate increases if they recommend and encourage a holistic approach.

Acupuncture

One of the main achievements of acupuncture is improving hemodynamics (blood circulation) to increase oxygen flow to the body's cells. Acupuncture opens up channels and redirects blood flow to areas that need it more. For example, when someone who suffers from back pain gets acupuncture to that area, the acupuncture needles target the channels in that area. Acupuncture improves the blood flow (perfusion), allowing better oxygen flow, decreasing or eradicating the pain over time. Blood, which serves as transportation of oxygen and other nutrients to the body, needs to have a smooth dynamic. Acupuncture improves this hemo (blood) dynamic. In doing so, it becomes a better transport to deliver other items required, such as hormones, proteins, and so on, to both the male and female reproductive organs.

Anderson and Rosenthal (2013) pointed out that "Due to the significant emotional and financial stress associated with undergoing IVF many women seek out other therapies to reduce stress levels and improve their IVF success rate." They stated that "Acupuncture is a common choice, partly because many randomized control trials (RCTs) investigating the impact of acupuncture on IVF has been undertaken."

Nola (Chapter 15) suffered devasting miscarriages and wanted to optimize her subsequent attempts. She heard about acupuncture and decided to use Google to find a place – she did. She explained that the day she walked into that acupuncture practice, her journey to motherhood shifted. Her subsequent pregnancy resulted in the birth of her happy, healthy son.

Acupuncture has become a desirable intervention by some physicians and patients over the past several years and is quite common in major cities and suburbs. As a result of relatively low success rate, high cost, and lack of or inadequate insurance coverage for traditional treatments, new therapies, including TCM that can improve pregnancy outcomes are used as adjunctive therapy for many and are on the rise.

According to Zheng, et al., (2014) "Although one trial has already reported that transcutaneous electroacupuncture stimulation (TEAS) significantly improved the clinical outcome of embryo transfer, stimulus frequency, treatment courses or times can be further optimized. Therefore, with appropriate intervention times (from the IVF injections phase) to the day of embryo transfer, enough treatment courses (six or seven sessions of acupuncture), syndrome differentiation and treatment according to individual characteristics, TEAS may produce a pleasantly surprising result."

Zheng et al. pointed out that in recent years, there have been a total of 23 randomized controlled trials evaluating acupuncture in IVF. These trials' latest comprehensive meta-analysis demonstrated acupuncture improved clinical pregnancy rate (CPR) among women undergoing IVF. Zheng further noted, "The difference was more distinct when the types of controls or different acupuncture times were examined in a sensitivity analysis. Acupuncture at approximately the same time as the stimulation/injection phase is more suitable than when performed only concurrently with egg retrieval or embryo transfer.

Many patients, of their own volition or testimonials from others, turned to complementary and alternative non-medical interventions to increase their conceiving success rate. Given that infertility results from reproductive issues, both men and women may benefit from acupuncture, herbs, etc., to reduce stress levels and increase blood circulation.

Studies show that those who receive even a small amount of these complementary treatments, such as acupuncture during an infertility cycle, are more likely to benefit from it because acupuncture improves the blood circulation to both uterus and ovaries. Overall, and from my own experience, acupuncture and massage therapy can significantly lower stress levels and improved relaxation and mental focus.

Herbs

Many herbs are on the market for every ailment possible as Western society tries to shift away from too many pharmaceuticals towards more natural remedies. Incorporating herbs into fertility care has increased. Studies show that herbs improve hormonal imbalance, decrease stress, and thereby impact fertility outcomes. It is especially critical that patients discuss herbal supplements with their infertility doctor and herbalist. These specialists must be aware of any contraindications between the infertility drugs and herbal supplements. Herbs can increase or counter the effect of pharmaceutical drugs and may potentially be unsafe. However, when both alternative and medical aspects are balanced and in harmony, the treatment successes will be at their best.

In her meta-analysis experiment, Karin Ried (2015) provided data from forty randomized control trials involving 4,247 women with infertility. The objective of this research was to "assess the effect of Traditional Chinese (herbal) Medicine (CHM) in the management of female infertility and pregnancy rates compared with Western medical (pharmaceutical) treatment" (Ried, page 116).

According to Ried, the study selection involved "RCTs with women of reproductive age with primary or secondary infertility. Infertility may have been associated with PCOS, anovulation, endometriosis, amenorrhea, Fallopian tube blockage, or unexplained causes. At the same time, the type of interventions included studies which used herbal medicine alone or in combination with Western Medicine (WM) in the form of drugs or surgery. The control group in RCTs received WM treatment only. The researchers excluded studies using acupuncture alone or TCM therapy combined with assisted reproductive technologies (ART).

The conclusion indicated that the CHM group's mean pregnancy rates were 60% compared with 33% in the WM group. This review suggested that managing female infertility with Chinese herbal medicine "improves pregnancy rates 2-fold within a 3-6-month period compared with Western medical fertility drug therapy only" (Ried).

Imagine if the western world incorporated this complimentary intervention more into their patients' care protocol how much their patients will succeed. Anderson and Rosenthal stated that "shorter duration of Chinese Medicine can be quite effective, especially in milder pathology cases of recent origin and may be relevant for women who have breaks between IVF cycles as an opportunity to incorporate the herbal benefits."

Massage Therapy

Massage therapy relaxes the body, mind, and emotions. Clients from all backgrounds and various needs find relaxation in massage, whether in a clinic or spa setting. In a research study conducted in 2015 (Okhowat, et al.) a research team's results suggested, "That undulation/massage therapy before blastocyst transfer improves embryo implantation, most likely due to a reduction in stress and elicits a relaxation effect on patients. These combinations reduce uterine contractions and enhance the blood flow in the abdominal region. For the optimization of IVF therapies, adjuvant therapies should be included as studies have shown their positive impact on pregnancy outcomes."

There are the cultural and religious barriers to be reckoned with in receiving alternative therapies such as acupuncture or taking herbs – these barriers must be respected by the clinicians. Susan Read et al (2014) shared an example of an Orthodox Catholic woman whose reliance on religious methods was intrinsically tied to her belief in the power of blessed talismans and her faith in the benevolence of patron saints of fertility.

Certain cultures do not embrace acupuncture, massages, and herbs. Some may have reservations about the western cultures and the methods they practice in aiding fertility because their practices are different. And some religions may also view fertility treatments as demonic.

Counseling

Failure to conceive brings emotional turmoil, especially to marriages and relationships. According to Karin Ried and Anne Alfred (2013), "Three-quarters (76%) of all women reported a high level of distress related to not having been able to have a child, and half of all women felt guilty or hurt when others made remarks about their childlessness. Coping techniques vary from drowning oneself in substance abuse to seeking religious and professional counseling."

These negative emotions had implications beyond personal identity and the relationship with the partner and often would influence social life and work relationships" (Ried and Alfred). Couples or individuals who seek counseling are best able to deal with the turmoil in a healthy way.

One of the most common coping strategies is venting. Some may vent to family, friends, clinicians, and just anyone. When couples are mistrustful or secretive about their issue, it is safer to vent in a counselor's office. However, according to Ried and Alfred, in a survey conducted in Australia, only one percent of clients took advantage of this service. Therefore, infertility nurses must be alert for signs of stress, identify them quickly, and offer suggestions for coping with the turmoil. Clinicians in the infertility world could be more alert to these cues so that they can discuss and recommend this therapy.

In their qualitative study, Fatemeh JafarzadehKenarsari et al. (2015) focused on supportive services and care based on the need for infertile couples' counseling needs. The study concluded, "Psychological counseling proved to be one of the significant needs of infertile couples. The experience of infertility imposes immense emotional distress on the individual and the couple, which can result in great social and psychological stress."

As a master's prepared registered nurse specialized in infertility, I recommend that the infertility healthcare system focuses on these evidence-based studies. Routinely incorporating a holistic approach would foster improved outcomes of infertility treatment. Patients and their partners would be more emotionally and psychologically cared for amidst the other pressing factors.

Nurses in this specialized field should improve their education related to contemporary and alternative medicine, provide that skill to patients, or refer them to specialty clinics for such adjunctive care upon embarking on fertility treatment. Based on evidence-based studies, this nursing care model will increase positive pregnancy outcomes and heal the emotional and psychological ailments and improve self-esteem. Regardless of whether an immediate positive pregnancy test or viable pregnancy results, when a patient receives holistic care, he or she will be able to handle the other challenges in a better way, and all else will improve.

Tips from an Infertility Nurse

Ask your provider about alternative therapy. Find a facility that specializes in treatment patients going through fertility treatment. Check with your insurance about coverage – some health plans include alternative therapies. Keep your fertility doctor posted on any herbal supplements or alternative therapies that you are taking.

Nola (Chapter 15) mentioned that she "heard" about acupuncture and decided to google searched to find her acupuncturist. You may need to do that too but if you are in the New York area, Holistic Medical in the New York City and South Shore Acupuncture & Fertility Wellness on Long Island, NY, are holistic centers that provides these therapies.

Chapter 25

Don't Go on This Journey Alone

You have been assigned this mountain
So that you can show others
It can be moved

— Mel Robbins

Approximately 4 million babies are born in the USA each year. Among them are over 75,000 births from assisted reproductive treatment (IVF & FET) including live births of about 8,500 from donor eggs or embryos cycles. Although over 280,000 ART cycles are performed each year in the USA (with some resulting in multiples) many cycles fail.

Infertility is real, and it strikes both men and women. When people are labeled "barren," the efforts to prove it wrong permeates every breath of their existence. The shock, stigma, shame, and guilt suddenly decrease a woman's worth and a man's ego, and the next breath is painful. The immediate impact is like being punched in the stomach. The pain exponentially increases as the individuals try to envision a future of not being able to have children.

It seems impossible to overcome severe infertility diagnoses such as no eggs, no sperm, or a defective uterus. While a woman or couple try to absorb the reality, the stress mounts, and the flood gates of the non-medical factors like dread, blame, uncertainty, and money matters rush in.

How do you handle this? Where do you start? Take a deep breath first and exhale. There is hope. First, acknowledge the grief this diagnosis brings and note grieving is the next step before moving forward. There is nothing wrong with letting this out through anger and tears. Then get up, roll up your sleeves, and go after the solution. Time may appear to move even faster, so let every minute count.

Talk to a trusted person other than your partner – this could be a relative, friend, religious leader, or counselor. Trying to explain to others what you are going through when they have never experienced the same situation may seem difficult and almost futile. Nevertheless, try to take the first step to talk to those you trust and know will support you in this journey even if they may not fully understand.

Talking softens the pain you feel inside and makes the journey more bearable, so talk about everything: medications, clinical procedures, fear, uncertainties, or marital difficulties. A support system keeps your sanity in place and saves marriages. Don't go on this journey alone – it becomes very lonely very quickly.

This book brings the reality of the diagnoses and the emotions. It also brings the solutions of various treatment protocols. This book includes the recommendations of alternative therapies to maximize the fullest potential of every effort to become a mom and dad. Put them all into perspective and find a reputable reproductive endocrinologist to move you through the journey. A second opinion is ok too if your instincts advise this.

The less aggressive fertility treatment options can be successful on the very first attempt but do not be discouraged if you must try again. For those who are not so lucky, remember if there is a tiny flicker of hope and the wildest chance of success at the next try, keep going and don't give up.

Having a baby with your own egg and sperm is what we know to be most natural, but it takes far more than this to make a baby. So, if you are out of eggs or sperm, remember that babies are made with more than those ingredients. They bring the added needed ones, which are an explosion of love, joy, fulfillment, sheer amazement, and an *eraser* for the stigma, shame, blame, and uncertainties.

As detailed in the patients' stories in Part Two, babies from a parent's own eggs and sperm did not subtract or add the true essence of a parent-child bond compared to babies born from a donor's eggs, sperm, embryos, and adoptions. Recent data indicates that over 140,000 children are adopted in the USA each year. The identity of gametes does not, and will not, negate the true embodiment of what a baby is to a mom and/or dad, or how the parents see and unconditionally love their children.

Each person has convictions and values, which dictate their ethics and choices. When being barren rips the fabric of your self-worth and destiny, anything gives. In the end, it behooves parents to do what is right for their children. If the child's DNA origin is different from that of the parent, find a way to disclose this information at an appropriate age of the child. Note: once the child is raised with love and emotional security, this task will be less daunting, and the bond may be even stronger and more respected. Do not risk breaking trust with your children in any circumstance, including how they were brought into this world and how they became your child. Trust is like glass. When broken, you cannot fully restore it.

And finally, remember that you are God's masterpiece. He created you after everything else and has given you the power to carry and nurture life inside and outside the body, and He will strengthen you to do this even amid difficulties if you let Him. Do not let the odds you face on this journey to parenthood keep you from doing what you know in your heart you were meant to do. Be a parent – love a child.

My Website: https://www.gentlenurse101.com

Some proceeds from this book will help some infertile couples who need it most.

Glossary

Abortion, Spontaneous — Pregnancy loss (miscarriage) by any cause before 20 weeks of gestation (pregnancy)

ACOG — American College of Obstetricians and Gynecologists - this is a professional association of physicians specializing in obstetrics and gynecology in the United States.

Adhesion — Scar tissue attached to internal organs such as the fallopian tubes, ovaries, uterus, or other internal organs. Adhesions can wrap up or distort these organs, limiting their movement and function and cause infertility and pain.

AMH - Anti-Mullerian Hormone — A hormone that measures egg reserve. A good AMH blood level is above 1.0 ng/ml.

Amniocentesis — A medical procedure done with ultrasound guidance in the second trimester of pregnancy to detect fetal abnormalities. It is performed by using a long sterile needle to withdraw a small quantity of the amniotic fluid that surrounds the fetus.

Aneuploidy — A condition of having a missing or extra chromosome. The risk of having a child with an aneuploidy increases as a woman ages. Trisomy (an extra chromosome in a fetus) is the most common aneuploidy.

Anonymous Egg Donor — A carefully-screened woman who is recruited specifically for egg donation to recipient couple and whose identities are kept confidential. These donors are compensated for the significant commitment of time and effort they make during the donation cycle.

Anonymous Sperm Donor	A man who confidentially donates his sperm to assist women to become pregnant whose identities are kept confidential.
ARA - Advanced Maternal Age	Advanced maternal age, in a broad sense, is the instance of a woman being of an older age at a stage of reproduction.
Aspermia or a zoospermia	The complete lack of semen with ejaculation, which is associated with infertility.
ASRM - American Society of Reproductive Medicine	Large multidisciplinary patient and physician organization serving as a platform for new ideas, education and advocacy in fertility and reproductive medicine issues. ASRM is a leading advocate for patient care, research, and education.
Assisted Reproductive Technologies (ART)	A group of fertility therapies that employ manipulations of the oocyte (egg) and sperm in the laboratory to establish a pregnancy. These include IVF, ICSI, donor egg cycles, assisted hatching, and preimplantation genetic screening.
Autologous Eggs	Eggs obtained from the same individual.
Basal Body Temperature (BBT)	The body temperature at rest taken in the morning before arising from bed. The daily reading is recorded and used to help identify the time of ovulation. This information is an especially important part of a BBT chart.
Biochemical Pregnancy	The absence of an identifiable pregnancy on ultrasound despite a positive urine or blood pregnancy test. This is referred to ask a chemical pregnancy as well. It occurs in the early pregnancy stage about 2-4 weeks from conception (soon after a missed period).
Cesarean (C-section)	Abdominal surgery to deliver a baby. The baby is taken out through an incision in the mother's abdomen.

Cervix	The lower section of the uterus which protrudes into the vagina and serves as a reservoir for sperm. Its anatomical functions include being a natural barrier to the inner uterus and keeping pregnancies from delivering prematurely.
Chorionic villus sampling (CVS)	Chorionic villus sampling (placental tissue) can reveal whether a baby has a chromosomal condition, such as Down's syndrome, as well as other genetic conditions, such as cystic fibrosis.
Chromosomes	Tiny components of cells that make organisms what they are. They carry all the information used to help a cell grow, thrive, and reproduce.
Clinical Pregnancy	A pregnancy in the uterus (womb) with beating fetal heart. This is identified by ultrasound.
Clomid (Clomiphene Citrate)	A medication in tablet form taken by mouth to stimulate the ovaries and/or synchronize follicle development.
COVID-19	COVID-19: "CO" stands for "corona". "VI" for "virus," and "D" for disease. Formerly, this disease was referred to as "2019 novel coronavirus" or "2019-nCoV". There are many types of human coronaviruses, including some that commonly cause mild upper-respiratory tract illnesses.
Cryopreservation	A controlled freezing procedure used to preserve human tissue such as sperm, embryos, and oocytes (eggs).
Cyst	A fluid-filled structure anywhere in the body. In the reproductive organ, these cysts are typically found on the ovaries - they can be normal or abnormal.

Cystic Fibrosis (CF) An inherited life-threatening disorder that damages the lungs and digestive system. Cystic fibrosis affects the cells that produce mucus, sweat, and digestive juices. It causes these fluids to become thick and sticky. They plug up tubes, ducts, and passageways.

Degenerate Whether used as a verb, noun, or adjective, degenerate carries a sense of making worse or declining to a lower state.

DES Exposure A large study of the daughters of women who had been given DES, the first synthetic form of estrogen, during pregnancy has found that exposure to the drug while in the womb (in utero) is associated with many reproductive problems and an increased risk of certain cancers and pre-cancerous conditions.

Diethylstilbestrol (DES) DES is a synthetic form of the female hormone estrogen prescribed to pregnant women between 1940 and 1971 to prevent miscarriage, premature labor, and related complications of pregnancy.

DNA - deoxyribonucleic acid DNA is the central information storage system of most animals and plants, and even some viruses.

Dominant Gene A dominant trait dominates the recessive ones. A dominant trait is an inherited characteristic that appears in an offspring if it is contributed from a parent through a dominant gene. Traits, also known as phenotypes, may include features such as eye color, hair color, immunity or susceptibility to certain diseases and facial features such as dimples and freckles.

Glossary

Donor Insemination — The introduction of sperm from an anonymous or known volunteer donor into the uterine cavity via the vagina/cervix to achieve a pregnancy. Donor sperm is also used in IVF to inseminate eggs in the fertilization process to make embryos.

Donor-egg IVF — The use of eggs (oocytes) donated by a someone (typically younger) to be used in an IVF procedure of a woman who cannot use her own eggs. These eggs are harvested via an IVF cycle performed on the donor. They are inseminated with sperm to form embryos which are transferred into the womb of the intended parent (recipient).

Donor-Embryo Transfer — The transfer of embryos that were formed from an egg and sperm of another patient. These embryos are donated by anonymous or known persons to an infertile recipient.

DOR - Diminished Ovarian Reserve — Diminished ovarian reserve (DOR) is characterized by poor fertility outcomes due to a decrease in egg quantity and quality, and it represents a major challenge in reproductive medicine.

Down's Syndrome — Down's Syndrome - a congenital disorder arising from a chromosome defect, causing intellectual impairment and physical abnormalities, including short stature, cardiac issues, and a broad facial profile. It arises from a defect involving chromosome 21, usually an extra copy (trisomy-21).

Ectopic Pregnancy A pregnancy that implants outside the uterus (womb), most often in the fallopian tube. This is also referred to as a tubal pregnancy. This is usually diagnosed in its early stages when the pregnancy hormone level is rising, but the pregnancy is not detected on ultrasound. It causes immense pain, and if left undiagnosed and untreated, can have serious medical consequences.

Egg Cryopreservation Cryopreservation of a woman's eggs is a freezing procedure to preserve her fertility. This technique has been used to enable women to postpone pregnancy to a later date – whether for medical reasons such as cancer treatment or for social causes such as employment, career development, or waiting for the right partner.

Egg Retrieval The procedure during an IVF cycle where the eggs are suctioned from the ovaries through a minimally invasive surgical procedure. This is done under light anesthesia so that patients are sleeping during the entire process. Typically takes about 20-30 minutes total.

Embryo The term used to describe the early stages of fetal growth - typically from conception to about 9 weeks.

Embryo Donation This is a form of third-party reproduction in which unused embryos remaining from one person/couple's successful In-Vitro Fertilization (IVF) treatment are donated to another person or couple. In most cases, this donation is anonymous. The donor parent/couple receives no money for donating the embryos, and the recipient does not pay for the embryos.

Embryo transfer	The procedure of transferring embryos back into the uterus of a patient during an IVF cycle. A fresh embryo transfer occurs on the third or fifth day after an egg retrieval. A frozen embryo transfer (FET) can be done any time after the embryos have been frozen.
Endocrinology	The study of hormones, their function, the organs that produce them and how they are produced.
Endometrial biopsy	The extraction of a small piece of tissue from the endometrium (lining of the uterus) for microscopic examination.
Endometrial Cavity	The space within the uterus that is created by an inner lining. This cavity responds to female hormones during the menstrual and treatment cycles. This lining, when properly prepared, forms the area of attachment and implantation of the embryo. The embryo grows in space until the time of birth.
Endometriosis	A disorder where the tissue that makes up the uterine lining (the lining of the womb) grows outside the uterus. Endometriosis is usually found in the lower abdomen or pelvis but can appear anywhere in the body.
Fallopian Tube(s)	The tubal structure that connects the uterus and the ovary, serves to transport the egg to meet the sperm to fertilize the egg. It is also this tube that the fertilized zygote (embryos) travels to the uterus for implantation.
FDA	Food and Drug Administration, a governmental agency involved in approving medications for use within the U.S. population.
Fertilization	The union of a sperm with an egg to facilitate creation of an embryo.

Fibroids	An overgrowth of the muscular tissue of the uterus. Fibroids are typically masses of benign muscle tissue that can distort the shape and function of the uterus. They can also hinder implantation of an embryo, and some, if problematic, may need to be removed before the woman attempts to get pregnant. Fibroids interfere with reproduction when they become severely enlarged or impinge on the uterine cavity.
Follicle	A fluid-filled pocket in the ovary that houses the microscopic egg. Follicles are often referred to as "egg nests". Each ovary has many follicles within it. Follicles start out extremely small and then grow larger under the influence of hormones or medications that mimic the function of hormones.
Follicle Stimulating Hormone (FSH)	Follicle Stimulating Hormone (FSH): A hormone produced by the pituitary gland in the brain that stimulates the ovarian follicles to grow and develop. FSH is measured in the blood at specialized times during the menstrual cycle to help measure ovarian reserve.
Gamete	A cell whose nucleus unites with that of another cell to form a new organism. A gamete contains only a single set of chromosomes.
Gamete Intrafallopian Transfer (GIFT)	In GIFT, the sperm and eggs (gametes) are mixed together before being inserted, and, with luck, one of the eggs will become fertilized inside the fallopian tubes.
Gestation	The process of carrying an embryo in the womb between conception and birth.
Gonadotropin Releasing Hormone (GnRH)	Gonadotropin Releasing Hormone (GnRH): Hormone produced by the hypothalamus in the brain that stimulates the pituitary gland to secrete gonadotropins.

Health Maintenance Organization	In the United States, a health maintenance organization is a medical insurance group that provides health services for a fixed annual fee. There are usually more restrictions with HMO insurance.
Heterosexual	This class of people is characterized by sexual or romantic attraction to or between people of the opposite sex (as in a male and female couple)
Human Chorionic Gonadotropin (hCG)	Human Chorionic Gonadotropin (hCG): A hormone of early pregnancy that is monitored to determine viability of the gestation. This hormone is also used as an injection to induce ovulation and maturation of the egg in ovarian stimulation protocols.
Hysterectomy	Hysterectomy is the surgical removal of the uterus. It may also involve removal of the cervix, ovaries, Fallopian tubes, and other surrounding structures.
Hysterosalpingogram (HSG)	A special x-ray procedure using a dye fluid to examine whether the Fallopian tubes are patent (open) or not. This test helps determine if there are blockages in the tubes that would prevent sperm from reaching the eggs.
Hysteroscopy	A minimally invasive surgery using a small telescopic camera placed into the uterine cavity via the vagina and cervix to allow direct visualization the inside of the uterine cavity (the womb). This surgical procedure is done under deep sedation and well-tolerated. It allows the removal of polyps, scar tissues, or fibroids in the uterine cavity that may hinder the implantation of an embryo.
Incompetent cervix	Also called a cervical insufficiency, occurs when weak cervical tissue causes or contributes to premature birth or the loss of an otherwise healthy pregnancy.

In-for-out (IFO)   In cases where there are only In-Network benefits, and the provider search reveals limited doctors, an insurance company may allow you to see an out-of-network doctor and pay as if the doctor/services were in-network.

In-Network (INN)   Your provider participates with your health insurance plan.

Infertility   The failure to achieve a clinical pregnancy after 12 months or more of regular unprotected sexual intercourse.

Insemination   The transfer of sperm into the uterus using a syringe with a plastic catheter. The purpose of insemination is to establish pregnancy.

Intracytoplasmic Sperm Injection (ICSI)   A procedure of injecting a single sperm into a single egg by penetrating the outer coatings of the egg. This technique is used in cases of abnormal semen analysis. ICSI is also used for patients who have had previous IVF cycles with failed fertilization and in fertilization of frozen eggs.

IUI - Intrauterine Insemination   Intrauterine insemination is an artificial insemination procedure. It is the deliberate introduction of sperm into a female's cervix or uterine cavity to achieve a pregnancy through in vivo fertilization by means other than sexual intercourse.

IVF - In-Vitro Fertilization	A more invasive procedure to help patients conceive pregnancies outside the body (in a lab). IVF involves the use of hormonal injections to stimulate a woman's ovaries to develop multiple follicles. When the eggs mature, they are harvested by the egg retrieval procedure, which is a surgical procedure under deep sedation for about 20-30 minutes. The eggs are then inseminated with sperm in the laboratory to create embryos that can then be transferred back to the endometrial cavity (the womb) of the patient 3-6 days later. The name in vitro fertilization refers to the fact that the sperm fertilize the egg in the laboratory, rather than inside the female reproductive tract.
Level II Ultrasound	This is an ordinary ultrasound done between 18-20 weeks of pregnancy and is like a standard ultrasound. The difference is that the doctor will get more detailed information. This ultrasound can detect structural anomalies such as cleft palate and genetic disorders such as spinal muscular atrophy.
LGBTQ	LGBTQ is an acronym for lesbian, gay, bisexual, transgender, and queer or questioning. These terms are used to describe a person's sexual orientation.
Menopause	The time of life when a woman's ovaries stop producing hormones and menstrual periods stop (typically between age 45-55).
Menses	A cyclic (monthly) flow of blood is also known as a "period" or "menstruation." It signifies ovulation but the absence of pregnancy. Onset of bleeding is considered cycle day 1. A natural menstrual cycle usually produces one follicle and ovulation per month, and when pregnancy is not achieved, the menses starts again.

Nuchal Translucency	This is a test done during pregnancy. It uses ultrasound to measure the thickness of the fluid buildup at the back of the developing baby's neck. If this area is thicker than normal, it can be an early sign of Down's Syndrome, trisomy 18, or heart problems.
Obstructive and Nonobstructive Azoospermia	There is a blockage or missing piece along the man's reproductive tract that hinders sperm production from exiting, so there is no measurable amount of sperm in the semen. *Nonobstructive azoospermia:* This type of azoospermia means the man has poor or no sperm production due to defects in the structure or function of the testicles or other causes.
Oocyte	An immature egg cell of the female ovary that matures during the menstrual cycle. When fertilized with sperm it becomes an embryo that becomes a baby.
Out-of-Network (OON)	Your provider does not participate with your health insurance plan.
Ovary	The female sex gland with both a reproductive function (releasing oocytes) and a hormonal function (production of estrogen and progesterone). A woman has two ovaries.
Ovidrel also called choriogonadotropin alfa	This is a drug given by injection to enhance and trigger ovulation. Ovidrel is also known as a "trigger shot." It may be used by itself or along with other fertility drugs.
Ovulation	The release of a mature egg from the ovary.
Ovulation Predictor Kit (OPK)	An OPK test is used to test when a woman is ovulating. It does not need a prescription. The test strip looks a pregnancy test strip but is designed to detect levels of luteinizing hormone (LH) in your urine. This hormone signals ovulation.

Pandemic	A pandemic is an epidemic occurring worldwide or over a very wide area, crossing international boundaries and usually affecting a large number of people.
Pituitary Gland	A small organ at the base of the brain that secretes many hormones, including LH and FSH in response to signals from the hypothalamus.
Placenta Abruption or Abruptio	A serious pregnancy complication in which the placenta detaches from the womb (uterus). The condition can deprive the baby of oxygen and nutrients. Symptoms include vaginal bleeding, belly pain, and back pain in the last 12 weeks of pregnancy.
Placenta Accrete	Placenta accrete is a serious pregnancy condition that occurs when the placenta grows too deeply into the uterine wall. Typically, the placenta detaches from the uterine wall after childbirth. With placenta accrete, part or all of the placenta remains attached. This can cause severe blood loss after delivery.
Placenta Previa	When the placenta covers the opening in the mother's cervix. The condition can also cause severe bleeding before or during delivery.
POF - Premature Ovarian Failure	A loss of normal function of the ovaries before age 40. POF is also referred to as "premature ovarian insufficiency (POI) and "early menopause".
Polycystic Ovarian Syndrome (PCOS)	A common endocrinologic condition that causes hormonal imbalances in women of reproductive age. It can lead to dysfunctional ovulation, infertility, weight gain, prediabetes, and an increase in the male hormone, testosterone.

Polyp An overgrowth of the glandular tissue on the surface of the uterine wall. Polyps like small bulbs of tissue that are often removed by hysteroscopy - a minimally invasive surgical procedure. If polyps are present, they can impede the implantation of an embryo on the wall of the uterus.

Preferred Provider Organization (PPO) PPOs offer participants much more choice for choosing when and where they seek health care. The biggest advantage that PPO plans offer over HMO plans is flexibility.

Preimplantation Genetic Diagnosis (PGD) Also referred to as PGT-m. A technique for identifying genetic or chromosomal information about embryos before transferring them back to a patient's womb to achieve pregnancy. It entails taking a biopsy of cells from the embryo on day three, five, or six after fertilization in the lab. PGD can be used to identify embryos that carry a genetic disease that may be a result of one or both parents being a carrier of a genetic mutation.

Preimplantation Genetic Screening (PGS) Also known as PGT-a. It is the screening for chromosomal abnormality. This screening determines if an embryo has more or less than 23 pairs of chromosomes. It also tells the gender of the embryo. Unlike PGD, PGS does not identify a genetic disease. PGS may be used to identify explanations for recurrent pregnancy loss and improve pregnancy outcomes in selected patients.

Progesterone	A hormone produced by the ovary which prepares the uterus for implantation and supports the early pregnancy. This hormone level also rises when ovulation takes place. If this hormone level is deemed to be inadequate during pregnancy, a progesterone supplement would be prescribed in the form of injections or vaginal suppository to support the early pregnancy.
Puberty	The period or age at which a person is first capable of sexual reproduction of offspring: in common law, presumed to be 14 years in the male and 12 years in the female.
Recessive Gene	Recessive is a quality found in the relationship between two versions of a gene. Individuals receive one version of a gene, called an allele, from each parent. In genetics, a trait that must be contributed by both parents to appear in the offspring. Recessive traits can be carried in a person's genes without symptoms of the disease.
Recurrent Pregnancy Loss (RPL)	The occurrence of three or more consecutive pregnancy losses. A pregnancy loss is defined as a clinically recognized pregnancy involuntarily ending before 20 weeks. A clinically recognized pregnancy means that the pregnancy has been visualized on an ultrasound or that pregnancy tissue was identified after a miscarriage.
Reproductive Endocrinologist	(RE) is the only type of medical doctor with specialized training focused solely on helping people become and stay pregnant. This doctor is also referred to as a fertility doctor.
Reproductive Endocrinology	Reproductive endocrinology and infertility are a surgical subspecialty of obstetrics and gynecology that trains physicians in addressing hormonal functioning as it pertains to reproduction as well as the issue of infertility.

Resolve.org	A nationwide non-profit organization established to promote reproductive health and to ensure equal access to all family building options for men and women experiencing infertility or other reproductive disorders.
SART - Society for Reproductive Technologies	The primary organization of professionals dedicated to the practice of IVF or assisted reproductive technology (ART).
Semen Analysis	Testing the male sperm sample under the microscope to determine sperm count, their ability to move forward (motility) and their shapes (morphology). The semen analysis is a cornerstone of the evaluation of couples experiencing infertility. The sperm count, motility and morphology all provide important information about how the sperm will perform in treatment cycles.
Sjogren's Syndrome	Sjogren's syndrome is an autoimmune disease that causes your immune system attack healthy cells instead of invading bacteria or viruses. Sjogren's also causes neuropathy (nerve pain) and can have a substantial risk of vaginal and cervical stenosis (narrowing).
Sperm	The smaller, usually motile male reproductive cell of most species that reproduce sexually.
Sperm Aspiration (TESA)	Testicular/Epididymal Sperm Aspiration (TESA): The removal of sperm directly from the testis or the epididymis using a needle for aspiration. This procedure is used for men who have no sperm in their ejaculates or have had vasectomies in the past. TESA is performed for ICSI.

Sperm Extraction (TESE)	Testicular/Epididymal Sperm Extraction (TESE): The surgical removal of sperm directly from the testis or the epididymis. Unlike "aspiration" as in TESA, a TESE is more like a biopsy procedure. This too is used for men who have no sperm in their ejaculates or have had vasectomies in the past. Sperm obtained through TESE also requires ICSI to ensure fertilization of the egg.
Sperm Capacitation	The physiological changes spermatozoa must undergo in order to have the ability to penetrate and fertilize an egg.
Spinal Muscular Atrophy (SMA)	A genetic disease affecting the central nervous system, peripheral nervous system, and voluntary muscle movement (skeletal muscle). Most of the nerve cells that control muscles are located in the spinal cord, which accounts for the word *spinal* in the name of the disease.
Surrogacy	Surrogacy is a method of assisted reproduction where intended parents work with a gestational surrogate who will carry for their baby(ies) in her womb until birth. Intended parents use surrogacy to carry their babies when they cannot do so on their own. Nowadays a surrogate is also referred to as a *gestational carrier*.
Testes (plural) and testis (singular)	Structures located in the scrotum to make sperm and testosterone (male hormone).
Timed Intercourse (TIC)	Timed intercourse is a simple treatment option for infertility. It involves monitoring your ovarian cycle via ultrasound and hormone testing and then having sexual intercourse around the time you are predicted to be most fertile.
Transvaginal Ultrasound	This is done by placing a probe through the vagina to visualize the portion of the female reproductive organs.

Tubal Patency	Lack of obstruction within the Fallopian tubes.
Ultrasound	High frequency sound waves that can be used painlessly, safely, and without radiation, to view the internal portions of the body. Ultrasound is especially useful for visualizing the female reproductive organs and pregnancies.
Unexplained Infertility	Inability to identify the cause of infertility despite a complete evaluation of male and female. In unexplained infertility, semen, ovarian reserve, ovulation, endocrinologic disorders and pelvic anatomy are all normal.
Urethra	The tube that connects the urinary bladder to the end of the urethra to remove urine. In men, the urethra carries semen also.
Uterus	Referred to as the womb, the uterus is the reproductive organ that houses, protects, and nourishes the developing embryo and fetus. It consists of the cervix, the endometrium (space in the womb), and the muscular layer that comprises the body of this reproductive organ.
Varicocele	A varicose vein around the ductus (vas) deferens and the testes. This may be a cause of low or no sperm counts, motility and morphology and lead to male infertility.
Vas deferens	The duct that carries sperm from the testicle to the urethra.
Zygote	The zygote is a fertilized egg. As it grows, it becomes an embryo and then at age 8 weeks is called a fetus.
Zygote Intrafallopian Transfer (ZIFT)	ZIFT is an infertility treatment used when a blockage in the fallopian tubes prevents the normal binding of sperm to the egg. Egg cells are removed from a woman's ovaries, and in-vitro fertilized. The resulting zygote is placed into the fallopian tube using a laparoscopic procedure.

CITATIONS

A limited market: the recruitment of gay men as surrogacy clients by the infertility industry in the USA. (2018). Retrieved from https://www.ncbi.nlm.nih.gov/pmc/articles/PMC6280596/

Anderson, B., & Rosenthal, L. (2013). Acupuncture and in vitro fertilization: Critique of the evidence and application to clinical practice. *Complementary Therapies In Clinical Practice*, 19(1), 1-5 5p. doi:10.1016/j.ctcp.2012.11.002

Ectopic Pregnancy. American Pregnancy Association. Retrieved from https://americanpregnancy.org/healthy-pregnancy/pregnancy-complications/ectopic-pregnancy-839.

FAQs. Early pregnancy loss. https://www.acog.org/womens-health/faqs/early-pregnancy-loss

Forman, E. (2020 April). Covid and IVF. https://www.youtube.com/watch?v=W8-jZbhntMw).

Gay Surrogacy – Surrogacy for the LGBT Couples. Retrieved from https://surrogate.com/about-surrogacy/types-of-surrogacy/can-lgbt-couples-pursue-surrogacy/

Gupta, S. (2017). Sjögren Syndrome and pregnancy: a literature review. *The Permanente Journal*, 21: 16-047. doi:10.7812/TPP/16-047

Hecker, A. (2020, April 15). What should I do with my unused embryos? Retrieved from https://www.nytimes.com/2020/04/15/parenting/fertility/ivf-unused-frozen-eggs.html

How Common is male infertility and what are its causes? Retrieved from https://www.nichd.nih.gov/health/topics/menshealth/conditioninfo/infertility.

Infertility Work-up for The Women's Health Specialists. (2019). Retrieved from https://www.acog.org/clinical/clinical-guidance/committee-opinion/articles/2019/06/infertility-workup-for-the-womens-health-specialist

Intended parents – surrogacy laws by state. Retrieved from https://surrogate.com/intended-parents/surrogacy-laws-and-legal-information/surrogacy-laws-by-state/

Jafarzadeh-Kenarsari, F., Ghahiri, A., Zargham Boroujeni, A., & Habibi, M. (2015). Exploration of the counseling needs of infertile couples: A qualitative study. *Iranian Journal of Nursing & Midwifery Research*, 20(5), 552-559. doi:10.4103/1735-9066.164506

Kruh, N. (2020, June 29). Baby joy after male infertility. *People*, 104.

Male Infertility. (2018). The American Pregnancy Association. Retrieved from https://americanpregnancy.org/infertility/male-infertility-70975.

Multiple Pregnancy and Birth: Twins, Triplets, and High Order Multiples. https://www.reproductivefacts.org/globalassets/rf/news-and-publications/bookletsfact-sheets

Okhowat, J., Murtinger, M., Schuff, M., Wogatzky, J., Spitzer, D., Vanderzwalmen, P., & Zech, N. H. (2015). Massage therapy improves in vitro fertilization outcome in patients undergoing blastocyst transfer in a cryo-cycle. *Alternative Therapies In Health And Medicine*, 21(2), 16-22.

Page, S, (2020, June 25). A woman is infertile, so her mother is carrying her baby. Retrieved from www.washingtonpost.com/lifestyle/2020/06/25

Perkins, K. et al, (2016, August). Trends and outcomes of gestational surrogacy in the United States, National Assisted Reproductive Technology Surveillance System (NASS) Group, *Fertility and Sterility*, Aug;106(2):435-442.e2. doi: 10.1016/j.fertnstert.2016.03.050. Epub 2016 Apr 14.

Picheta, R. (2020, November 25). Meghan, Duchess of Sussex, reveals she had a miscarriage in July. https://amp-cnn-com.cdn.ampproject.org/c/s/amp.cnn.com/cnn/2020/11/25/uk/meghan-sussex-miscarriage-oped-scli-intl-gbr/index.html.

Premature Ovarian Failure (POF. Resolve.org). Retrieved from https://resolve.org/infertility-101/medical-conditions/premature-ovarian-failure.

Read, S. C., Carrier, M., Whitley, R., Gold, I., Tulandi, T., & Zelkowitz, P. (2014). Complementary and alternative medicine use in infertility: cultural and religious influences in a multicultural Canadian. https://www.ncbi.nlm.nih.gov/pmc/articles/PMC4155414/

Reproductive Health, Infertility FAQs. Retrieved from https://www.cdc.gov/reproductivehealth/infertility/

Ried, K. (2015). Chinese herbal medicine for female infertility: an updated meta-analysis. *Complementary Therapies In Medicine*, 23(1), 116-128 13p. doi:10.1016/j.ctim.2014.12.004

Ried, K, & Alfred, A. (2013). Quality of life, coping strategies and support needs of women seeking Traditional Chinese Medicine for infertility and viable pregnancy in Australia: a mixed methods approach. *BMC Women's Health*, 13(1), 1-11. doi:10.1186/1472-6874-13-17.

Sechtin, D. (2020, November 19). Embryo frozen 20 years ago becomes Louisville couple's snowflake baby, retrieved from https://www.whas11.com/article/life/heartwarming/embryo-adoption-snowflake-baby-frozen

Shapiro, C. (2010, August 20). New research on stress and infertility. [Web log post]. Retrieved from https://www.psychologytoday.com/us/blog/when-youre-not-expecting/201008/new-research-stress-and-infertility

Shapiro, D. (2019). *Inheritance.* Penguin Random House.

Shepherd, G. (2020, September 09). What does it all mean - PGT-A, PGT-M, and PGT-SR. [Web log post]. Retrieved from https://ormgenomics.com/2018/09/20/pgt-what-does-it-all-mean/

Shriver, Eunice Kennedy. (2020). About Endometriosis – NICHD. Retrieved from https://www.nichd.nih.gov/health/topics/endometriosis

Steussy, L. (2019, March 29). This grandma just gave birth to her own granddaughter. Retrieved from https://nypost.com/2019/03/29/this-grandma-just-gave-birth-to-her-own-granddaughter/

Strohm, E. (2020, October 5). Comedian Michele Buteau: An overnight success….after two decades. *People.* 73

Sumner, J. A goodbye letter to my embryos. [Web log post]. Retrieved from https://pregnantish.com/a-goodbye-letter-to-my-embryos-by-jamie-sumner/

Surrogacy laws in New York. Retrieved from https://www.circlesurrogacy.com/surrogacy/surrogacy-by-state/surrogacy-in-new-york

The ZyMot Multi (850) sperm separation device. Retrieved from https://zymotfertility.com/products/zymot-multi-850%c2%b5l

Turocy, J., Robles, A, Hercz, D., D'Alton, M., Forman, E., Williams, Zev. (2020, August). The emotional impact of the ASRM guidelines on fertility patients during the Covid-19 pandemic. *Fertility and Sterility.* doi: 10.1016/j.fertnstert.2020.08.194

Webster, A. and Schuh, M. (2016, October 20). Mechanisms of aneuploidy in humans. *Trends in Cell Biology*, DOI: https://doi.org/10.1016/j.tcb/2016.09.002.

Wenn, (2006, November 14). Crosby dismayed about donating sperm to Etheridge. Retrieved from https://www.contactmusic.com/david-crosby/news/crosby-dismayed-about-donating-sperm-to-etheridge

Zheng, C. H., Zhang, J., Wu, J., & Zhang, M. M. (2014, May 09). The effect of transcutaneous electrical acupoint stimulation on pregnancy rates in women undergoing in vitro fertilization: a study protocol for a randomized controlled trial. *Trials*, 15:162. doi:10.1186/1745-6215-15-162

CONSIDER WRITING A REVIEW

When you enjoy a book, it is a natural desire to tell others about it. Amazon and other online book sale platforms provides a way to share your thoughts and I invite you to write a book review. It is easy. Here are tips:

1. After going to your preferred platform, the first thing you are asked to do is to **assign a number of stars** to the book that matches your opinion of the book.

2. Create a **title** for the review. This can be a simple phrase, like "Awesome book." If you are not sure what to say, look at the titles of other book reviews.

3. It is easiest to write the book in a **word processor** and then paste it into Amazon.com. Your word processor will pick up typos before your review goes public.

4. Write the review as if you were **talking to another person** – you are – a person who comes to the website and is considering buying this book.

5. Include a description of what you found **most helpful**. Was it an idea, chapter, tip? Share that with the readers.

6. Next you may want to write **who you think would most benefit** from this book. Is it for infertile cou-

ples or their families? Or is it more appropriate for some - one with experience with this topic?

7. What if you have something **negative** to say about the book? You may always reach me at prasheed1@icloud.com to suggest changes in the book.

8. If you include negative feedback in the review, keep a positive perspective rather than attack me.

Here are some sample phrases:

- While overall the book was good, I would change it by. . .
- I don't think this book is right for. . .
- I would improve this book by. . .

Before you hit save, **read everything over one more time**. Authors and readers appreciate book reviews and they get easier to write with time.

Also please email me at prasheed1@icloud.com when you have posted your review.

Thank you,

Pamela Rasheed

www.ingramcontent.com/pod-product-compliance
Lightning Source LLC
Chambersburg PA
CBHW060823220526
45466CB00003B/951